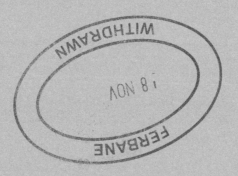

# VOGUE WILLIAMS

## everything

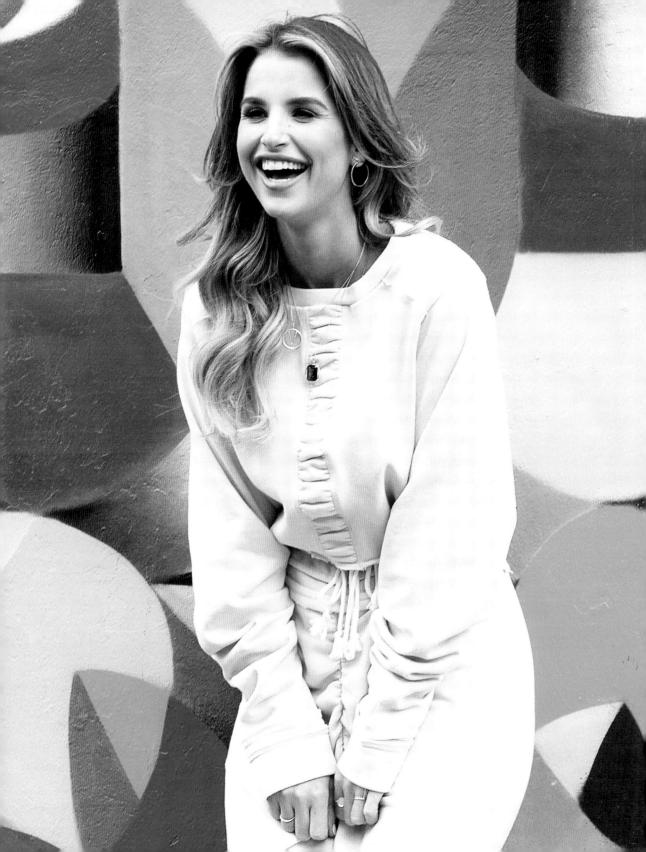

# VOGUE WILLIAMS

*everything*

## BEAUTY. STYLE. FITNESS. LIFE.

HACHETTE
BOOKS
IRELAND

First published in 2017 by Hachette Books Ireland
An Hachette UK Company

1

ISBN: 9781473649323

Typeset in Akzidenz Grotesk by Anú Design, Tara
Book text design by Anú Design, Tara
Cover design by Head Design
Printed and bound in Germany by Mohn Media GmbH

Hachette Books Ireland policy is to use papers that are natural, renewable and recyclable products
and made from wood grown in sustainable forests. The logging and manufacturing processes are
expected to conform to the environmental regulations of the country of origin.

Hachette Books Ireland
8 Castlecourt Centre
Castleknock
Dublin 15
Ireland

A division of Hachette UK, Carmelite House, 50 Victoria Embankment, London EC4Y 0DZ, England
www.hachettebooksireland.ie

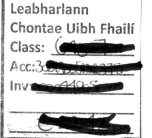

*I would like to dedicate my book*
*to my amazing mother Sandra.*
*She is the person I admire most in the world*
*and it would take me lifetimes to repay her*
*for everything she has done for me.*
*This dedication is my way of apologising*
*for those 'monster years' I went through as a teenager.*

# Contents

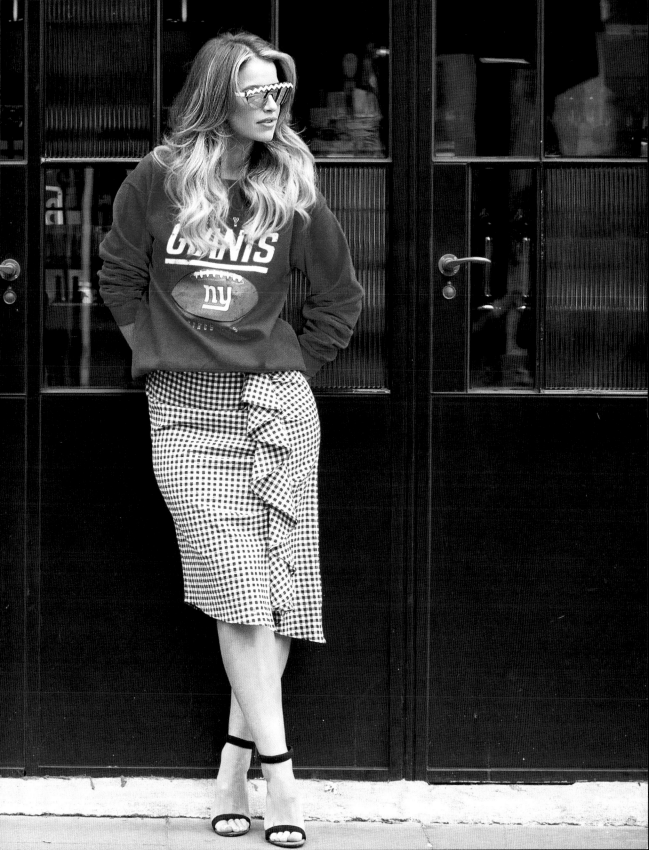

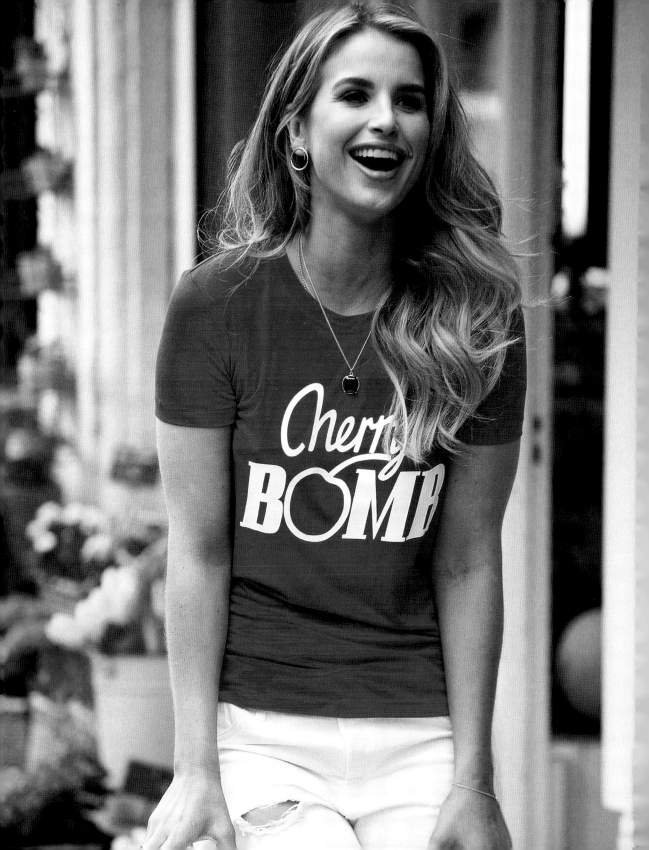

# Introduction

I can't believe that I am writing the introduction to my book – 'surreal' doesn't quite describe it.

I like to set myself goals every New Year's Eve – I'm not into resolutions; I think a goal is way better – and in 2016 my goal was to write a book. I always wanted to do a lifestyle-type book because I believe that it's important to be healthy and happy but also that introducing and maintaining positive changes in your life shouldn't have to take up all of your time.

We all lead fast-paced lives and, sometimes, we push the things that make us truly happy to one side because of work or other obligations. Even though I love my job and everything I do, I can sometimes put work before other areas of my life that I know should take priority.

I want to share with you the things I do to ensure that I can do my job well, keep fit and eat healthily while still leaving time to relax, have fun and spend time with my family and friends. I like to enjoy everything I can in life – whether it's eating a pizza, going on a shopping spree, spending the whole day in bed or going to work – but having fun and being healthy doesn't have to be an either/or situation. They can go hand in hand, and prioritising both is essential for my happiness – and yours.

Making time for everything is important to me, but it can be difficult. A lot of what I do involves preparation and planning. I'm all about efficiency and making the most of my time, so I'll always opt for intense thirty-minute gym sessions over being there for hours, or spending one afternoon making my weekly meals rather than cooking every evening after a long day. But it has taken a bit of experimentation to figure out what works best for me.

When it comes to food, I pay a lot of attention to how healthy my meals are, but they also need to taste good. I'm a big foodie. Often when I'm munching on my avocado and toast at breakfast, I'm already thinking about what I'm going to have for lunch or dinner. Dieting has never appealed to me, but I have changed the way I eat over the years and have a lot of yummy go-to recipes in my arsenal. I've included some of my favourites in this book as well as some of my healthy-ish cocktails – we all need to let loose every so often!

Feeling good on the outside is also important. Having a healthy relationship with your body can be tough and being comfortable in my own skin is something I'm working on all the time. But I find that what I wear can be an important part of it for me. It allows me to express myself, and an outfit that makes me feel good – because it's flattering or because it has good memories attached to it or maybe it's just a colour I love – can lift my mood on a day where I'm not feeling the best.

I do think some people are born stylish – I'm pretty sure Olivia Palermo came out of the womb wearing Chanel – and others might have more to spend on their wardrobe, but I do think style can be achieved by anyone. It's all about enhancing your figure, having fun with fashion and making sure you wear clothes that feel like you. I'm really excited to share my style tips in this book.

We all have so much on our plates – and our minds – these days: work, family, keeping fit, eating right and making time for the people we love and for self-care. It's important for me to take this holistic approach to health, making sure I'm doing everything I can to feel good, inside and out. And working hard feels so much more worth it when I can also take the time to really enjoy life. I'm not an expert on fitness or beauty but I've learned a lot through the years, so in this book I'm sharing with you the things I do to achieve this balance – I hope you like it!

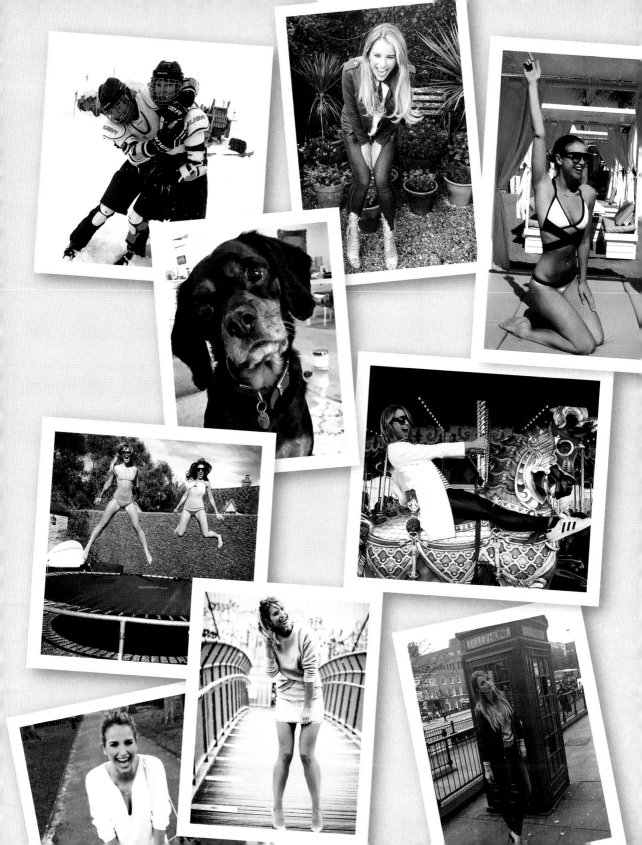

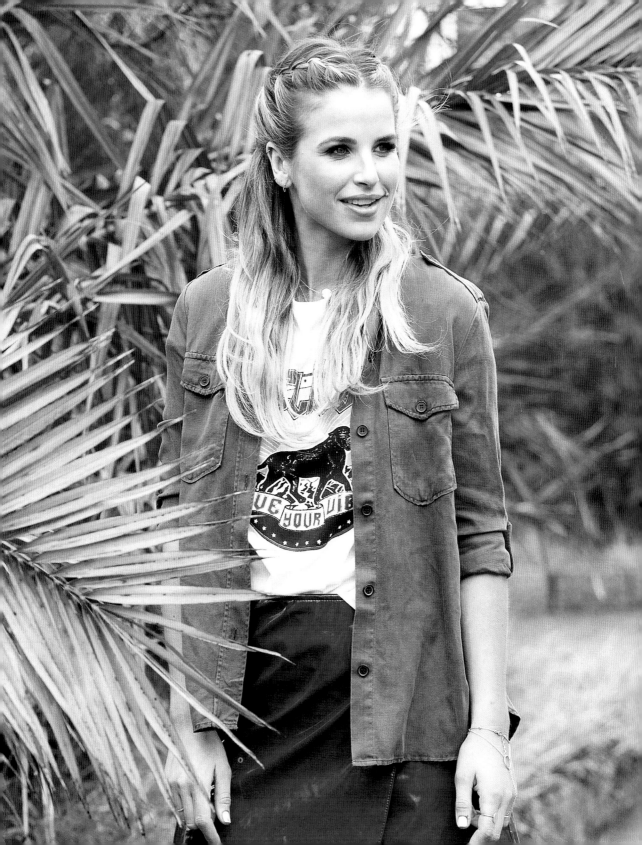

# About Me

I was born in Dublin on 2 October 1985 and spent the first seven years of my life living in Portmarnock, a quiet suburb not too far from Dublin city centre, with my mom, Sandra, my dad, Freddie, and my older brother and sister, Frederick and Amber.

My parents separated when I was seven. I don't remember being particularly upset by it at the time but now I see that it probably affected me more than I knew. My parents' split wasn't amicable and my dad acted in ways he shouldn't have, something I know he realised in later life. My brother and sister remember more about that time in our lives and, after hearing their stories, I'm glad this isn't true for me.

The years that followed my parents' break-up were difficult, especially for my mom – I honestly don't know how she did it, and if I think about it too much I get upset because of what she went through. We were never poor but we weren't rich either. My mom worked incredibly hard as a single mother to give us what we needed. She was an air hostess with Aer Lingus and also waitressed to support us. I wasn't rolling around in the latest Nikes but when we picked up a new hobby, of which there were many, my mom always made sure we were able to go for it regardless of what it cost. When my friends and I started playing hockey, Mom managed to get about ten old hockey sticks for us from my aunt, who was a teacher and had some left over in school. That's the way my mom is – resourceful and selfless. Even when she had it really tough, she made sure we didn't notice. And I'm sure bringing up three children alone wasn't easy, especially because my sister and I were such messers – Frederick is the eldest and was definitely an easier child to deal with. My mom is the strongest woman I know. She

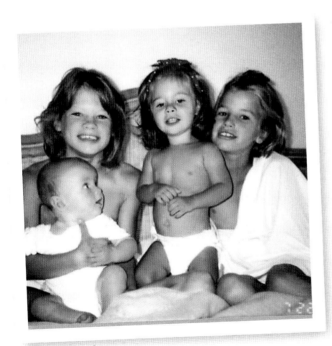

I'm a real family person.

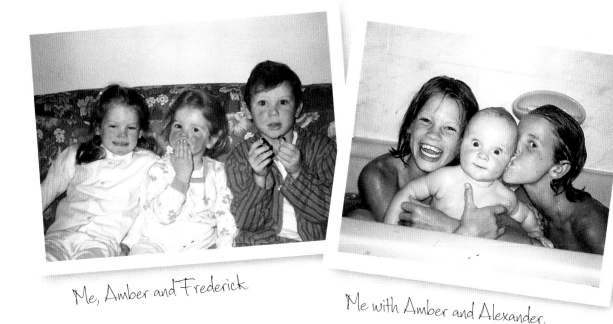

Me, Amber and Frederick.

Me with Amber and Alexander.

is always up for a laugh and is a really hard worker. She is an incredible person who I admire so much.

My dad lived close by and took us out on Wednesdays after school and every second weekend, which he never missed. Sometimes he would come to our school during lunch break and give us a Brunch and a Snickers each through the gates. We were big fans of this routine, and the Brunch is still my favourite ice-cream, despite my mom jokingly telling me that the crumbly bits on the outside had been swept up off the ground (she didn't like my expensive taste in ice-creams).

I was around eight years old when my mom met Neil, who became my stepdad. And shortly afterwards we moved to Howth, my favourite place in the whole world, to live with him. I didn't feel anything strange about it – I was given some new Play-Doh so I was quite happy to move if it meant getting presents.

Around three years after my mother and Neil got married, my glorious little brother Alexander was born, though I did not take the news well at first. I didn't like the idea of not being the youngest anymore, but when my mom told me I could use his clothes for my dolls, I perked up. Alexander became my real-life doll and I loved looking after him. He slept in my bed with me until he was about five and we spent a lot of time together as children. My little brother is probably the best-behaved out of the four of us, the golden child, closely followed by Frederick.

I'm a real family person and my siblings are my best friends, although we did have occasional (ahem, loads of!) fights when we were younger. I used to share a bedroom with Amber and if I took any of her stuff there'd be trouble. She also used to make up songs and force me to perform them! But once I accepted that she was in charge then it was all fine. Though I can recall hitting her with a plank of wood at one of her birthday parties – that was nice of me!

Frederick was a bit cooler than my sister and me, and he was always off with his mates, though we were still close. But Amber and I have always been best friends. We spent some of our childhood picking chewing gum off the ground and eating it or smoking the ends of cigarettes we found on the street together – I'm glad we've since given up those two things!

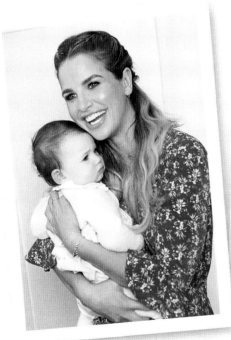

My niece Jeanie.

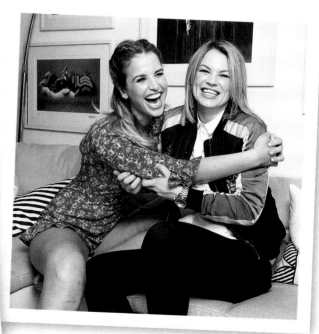

Me and my sister, Amber.

When we were very young, Amber and I loved to make 'agendas' filled with what we would do at the weekend. One of our favourite things to do was to borrow our neighbours' clothes and go and swim in the swamp – a huge pond near where we used to live. We were little tomboys but smart enough not to wreck our own clothes for fear of getting into trouble so borrowed our neighbours' instead, their mom didn't mind! I am still a big planner – it's something my friends always make fun of me about, but I just can't help myself. A day without a plan is an uneasy day for me – I always prefer to know what I'm going to be doing!

Neil, whom I view as a second father, was quite strict – actually, that's a lie: he was insanely strict, though Amber and I were brats so I guess he had to be. He's Scottish and does enjoy the odd screech at an unruly child. He was also generous and he made sure that we had an amazing childhood, but swearing in front of him is something that can still get me in trouble, even at the age of thirty-one.

As I grew older, my relationship with my dad became a lot more difficult. My mom and Neil didn't like me speaking about him at home, and I always felt like they were annoyed with me when I came home from one of our visits. Now I understand why they disliked him so much, but at the time it was hard to feel caught in the middle. I know they were being protective, but I wanted to stay close to my dad too.

I didn't help things by sneaking off to discos with my friends, when my mom had told me I couldn't go. I did things like that quite a lot, so much so that my mom and Neil kicked me out when I was seventeen. I went to live with my dad for a year and had no contact with Mom or Neil. This was a very tough time for me because I am so close to my mom, though I did enjoy living with my dad – I certainly got to take more time off school.

Looking back, I can see I was more affected by what happened with my family than I thought at the time. So much was changing and while some of the changes were great – such as the arrival of my little brother – it was a lot to handle at times. I know now that my mom and Neil had my best interests at heart, but we weren't able to communicate properly and this led to argument after argument which looking back was mainly my fault. I think that when you're a teenager it's very hard to sit and talk to your parents about how you feel. I loved my dad very much but felt lonely being away from the rest of my family while I was living with him. I'm very close to my aunt Naomi and talking to

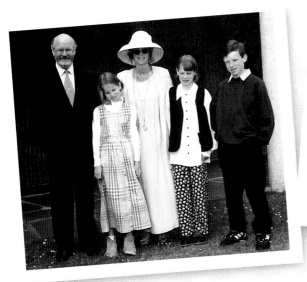

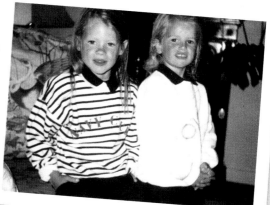

Me and Amber.

I obviously get my love of hats
from my mom.

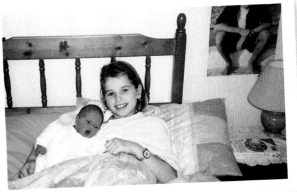

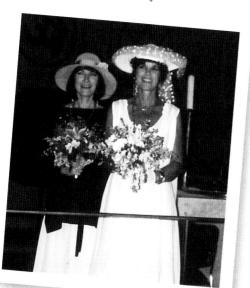

Me with Alexander.

Naomi and my mom
on her wedding day.

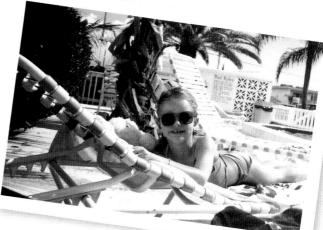

6

Always sunglasses and a bikini.

her was such a help to me during that time. And that's the advice I would give to young people going through their parents' separation – find someone understanding to talk to about what's going on.

Although I often tried to bunk off school, I did like it, but I wasn't very well behaved. I figured out how to forge my parents' signatures, all three of them, so when the mood would take me I'd leave school at lunchtime, note in hand about a fictional dentist's appointment or important family trip. I'd go down to the beach with a friend and just hang out. And my inability to stop talking got me suspended twice but I guess it has served me well in my adult life!

My favourite memories of my time at secondary school involve my friends. My best friends then – Ashley, Clodagh and Sarah – are still my best friends now. As teenagers, we spent all our time together. At school, we would pass notes to each other and gossip at lunchtime, making plans for the weekend. Weekends consisted of stealing alcohol from our parents, then hanging out around our area and drinking (I still don't know if my mom knows that I did that – well, she does now!).

But, unlike my friends, I wasn't allowed out after school during the week. So I spent a lot of time at home, mostly babysitting my little brother. My family lived in an amazing house in Howth which had a tennis court and swimming pools, a big change from what we'd been used to before. So, though sometimes I felt I was missing out on fun with my friends, I definitely appreciated having such a nice place to go home to in the evenings.

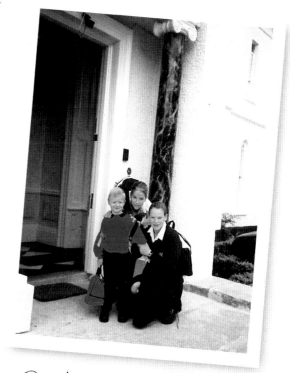

*Outside our home in Howth.*

I started modelling when I was sixteen, which I was allowed out for. Modelling wasn't something I had ever thought about doing when I was younger – it wasn't a long-held passion. I was just spotted leaving a hairdresser's in town by a talent scout and that was that. The first shoot I did was for a hair show. I didn't really see it as a career at first – myself and my friends weren't really thinking about college and careers at that stage, and I wasn't quite sure what I wanted to do – so I saw it more as a source of fun. I was learning about hair and make-up, getting to wear stylish clothes, meeting new people. And earning my own money made me feel more independent.

I do remember feeling quite young on one of my first shoots, which was for

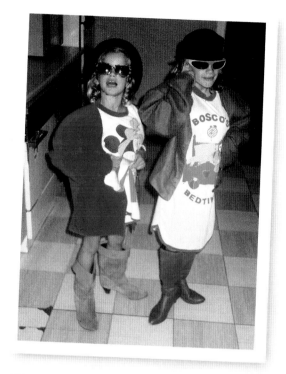

*I was into sunglasses and boots from a very young age.*

wedding dresses. I was very quiet because I didn't want to cause any trouble. The dress I was modelling was tiny so I had to be squeezed into it, and I was absolutely roasting under all the lights. I was also too embarrassed to ask for lunch, so I continued with the shoot only to faint after an hour. I never made that mistake again! That said, in Ireland, I never felt under any pressure from the industry to skip meals or lose weight.

I loved those early years of modelling. I got to do the most ridiculous photocalls – yes, I was the girl in Stephen's Green in my bikini – but it was always a laugh. I did intend to go to university: I planned to continue with my modelling career while studying architecture at Trinity College. My brother had studied architecture, Neil was a property developer and I loved programmes like *Grand Designs* so it seemed a natural thing for me to do – but I hadn't considered that I would need to study hard! By the time of my final year in school, I had moved back home and, unfortunately, 'studying' meant either sleeping with a book over my face in case my mom came in or writing stacks of notes to my friends during after-school study sessions. The day the Leaving Cert. results came out wasn't a great one for me – I hadn't achieved the grades I had hoped for, so the university courses I wanted weren't an option. I remember feeling really disappointed, especially as I saw my friends' delight about getting the courses they'd applied for. While, of course, a lot of people do well without exam success, I do regret sometimes that I didn't try my best. Maybe that's part of the reason why I'm such a hard worker now! However, as was my way at the time, I brushed it off, deciding I would do a course that would get me into college the following year instead, and off I went to celebrate with my friends. I could make plans for, and worry about, the future later.

But after three days my celebrations – and burying my head in the sand – came to an abrupt end. Neil had an ultimatum: I had to either move out and get a job to pay my way, or go to university in Aberdeen to study construction design and management, one of the few courses I'd been accepted for. And he had already booked a flight to Scotland. I didn't want to leave Dublin, and my friends and family, behind – but I felt I had no choice. I wasn't going against my parents' wishes again.

And, though it was difficult at times, I ended up enjoying my time in Aberdeen. I moved into student accommodation and had great fun living with my flatmates. And I made a lot of friends, including Ricky, who I'm still good mates with. He lives in London now and he's one of the funniest people I know.

Aberdeen was a great student city, and I went out to gigs a few nights a week. I saw a lot of my favourite DJs there, and I don't think I would have ended up DJing myself if it hadn't been for that. I also worked in a bistro-type restaurant and made a lot of new friends there who loved the same music as me – it wasn't rare for us to start drinking in work (on the sly) at around 10 p.m. so we'd be ready for our night out when our shift had finished.

I had a couple of fleeting romances in college but nothing long-term or serious. That was until I met my first love, Al, in Dublin. I was going into my final year in Aberdeen but had been working as a promotional waitress at home during the summer. I wasn't a great waitress and there was an incident with a tray (which I won't go into!) the night I met Al at an event. We hit it off the moment we saw each other but then later in the night I ended up being fired. When I went up to Al and told him what had happened, he asked for my number. We had an up-and-down relationship over the next six years – especially when we were dating long distance – and we didn't speak for a few years after we broke up, but now he is one of my closest friends and someone I place a lot of trust in. He gives me advice on a daily basis!

As part of my college degree I had to work in London for six months as a site engineer. I realised quite quickly that working on a building site wasn't for me, mostly because it was usually freezing! My boss allowed me to pick my own steel-toe-capped boots and jacket as little bribes to get me on site, but it didn't make me enjoy the experience any more! I was interested in what I was studying – and I was getting good results in my exams – but being on site made me wonder if I was really where I was supposed to be, if this degree was going to lead me to a career I enjoyed. I sometimes wish I had planned more carefully for what I would do when I finished school, but it's not always easy to figure that out when you're a teenager.

I liked Aberdeen but, for me, the main problem was that it was a bit too far out of the loop in terms of modelling and DJing and everything I knew I really wanted to do. However, at the end of the day, I had some fantastic experiences there, and everything I've done in my life has led me to where I am now. That's the attitude I prefer to take – all of my experiences have made me who I am, and I've learned lots along the way.

I moved home to Dublin after finishing my degree and decided to continue on my chosen career path by studying Quantity Surveying at the Dublin Institute of Technology. Even though I'd already been having second thoughts about this being the career for me, I was conscious that my parents had given me a lot of help with my education and it was important to them, so I didn't want to let them down. I went straight into the second year of the Dublin course, because I already had my degree, which was hard because everyone already knew one another. I did make friends, though, as with Aberdeen, there were few girls on this course, so my friends were mainly boys. It was while I was studying at DIT that I felt bullied for the first time in my life, and it made that period of adjustment much harder than it should have been.

One of the girls in my class took an instant dislike to me, and it felt like she was constantly making an effort to exclude me, which was really hurtful. But I did my best

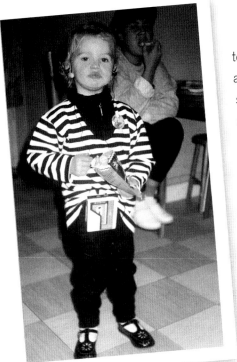

*Always into my music!*

to ignore her behaviour and her negativity and get on with my studies. Bullying is such a difficult, painful experience and I really hope that anyone reading this who is being bullied asks for the help they need. Sometimes people bully others because they themselves are in terrible pain, but it's tough to keep this in mind when you are the one being singled out and the object of their anger or cruelty. Remember that no one has the right to make you unhappy –

to take away your enjoyment and feelings of safety at school or college, in your workplace or even in your home. And being different is never a bad thing, though, unfortunately, there are people who will try to make you feel as though it is. Please don't go through it alone – talk to someone you can trust. I know talking about it really helped me a lot.

Overall, though, I was happy to be back in Dublin because it was easier to keep up with my modelling, while keeping my parents satisfied by getting another degree. I also began DJing professionally

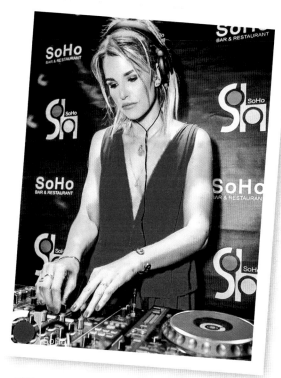

*I began to DJ professionally when I moved back to Dublin.*

11

when I moved back. I had a manager who worked for MCD music promotions and I started doing a lot of sets in clubs.

However, I began to realise that what I really loved was media, and television in particular. I'd always dreamed of working in TV but hadn't thought it would be possible to pursue as a career. I definitely had the gift of the gab and as a child I regularly pretended to conduct interviews in our kitchen. I also felt modelling had given me a confidence I wouldn't have had otherwise to put myself out there and cope better with the ups and downs of a media career.

Just as I was gathering the courage to tell my parents about my feelings, the building industry collapsed, making my current career path more unstable. Despite this, I was nervous talking to them about my plans, but they were really supportive. Neil told me recently that they didn't know how to help me get into a career in television, and that's why they were wary of it. The whole idea of a career in the media was quite a foreign concept to them. I really look up to my stepdad, I always have, he's so great in business and I definitely wanted to make him proud. Now, he tells me all the time how proud he is of what I'm doing and what I achieve, and he watches everything I do!

I suppose my first break was being in *Fade Street* in 2010, a reality show inspired by MTV's *The Hills*. It was fun to be part of, though I realised quite quickly that reality TV wasn't where I wanted to be. I didn't like my private life being in the public eye and it was loosely scripted, which I didn't like either.

I was still with my boyfriend Al when we were filming the show and he definitely didn't want to be involved in it. The producers kept trying to get one of the guys to flirt with me, to create some excitement for the show, and that started to mess with my off-screen, real life. I like a drama-free, easy life but never seem to have one. But even though there were difficult moments, I certainly don't regret doing the show – I made a lot of friends and had great fun.

After I finished *Fade Street* in 2011, I got a presenting gig for a one-off programme – *Vogue Does Home and Away* – about the Australian soap that's hugely popular in Ireland. I went to Australia to film it and met a lot of the *Home and Away* cast, and the programme got a great reaction from the public, leading to another presenting job. But the hours were long, so I didn't get to see much of the country, though I solved that by eventually moving there for two years.

In 2011, just as my career was blossoming in Ireland, I met Brian McFadden. At the time he was promoting his third solo album and was back and forth between Ireland and Australia. We got very serious very fast and, only a few weeks into our relationship, I decided to move to Australia with him. We got married in 2012.

Though going to Australia was a bit of an impulsive decision, I have never regretted it. The move happened shortly after my dad's death, a really difficult time in my life, and now I can

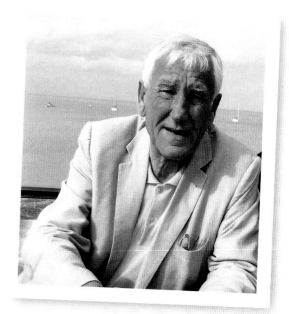

My dad.

see that I was running away from my sadness and pain. I didn't want to be at home, where everything reminded me of my father, because I was too busy trying to pretend he hadn't died. Dad's death still haunts me; I still feel like I only saw him yesterday. I can remember his voice and his smell, but I worry that there will come a time when I won't be able to remember these things.

Growing up, my dad was always quite sick. He lived 'the good life' and was fond of cigarettes and drink. Add putting butter on your chips and that was him! He had two heart attacks when I was very young and I remember being brought to see him in the hospital but I wouldn't look at him – it was too scary. He had a triple bypass, a stroke and other ailments over the years but didn't complain too much about any of it. Immediately after his first stroke, when I was twenty-one, he wasn't able to speak and half of his body was paralysed, but miraculously, after a week, he suddenly went back to his old self, and we all relaxed. However, four years later, he discovered that he had an aneurysm in his stomach that needed an operation, which was very risky – it was the first time I saw fear in my dad's eyes.

I honestly thought he would be fine. I was worried, but he was my dad and he always pulled through. I remember the day he went in for the operation and I also remember my joy at hearing he had got through it, so I went straight in to the hospital to see him. When I got to his room, I thought he was acting quite strangely – he wasn't saying the sort of things he would usually say – but the doctors assured me he was fine, so I went home. However, his condition slowly worsened over the next few days. Then he had another stroke and was in a coma.

Myself, my sister and my aunt had to meet with the surgeon to decide what to do next and whether or not we should turn off Dad's life-support machine. I didn't want to – I wanted to give him more time to fight – but, in hindsight, that was selfish. He would have had no quality of life if my sister and Aunt Sharon had not made the decision to let him go. It was six o'clock on a Friday morning when I watched my dad die as I held his hand. I could see the life leave him and then he was gone. It just can happen so quickly – suddenly, that's it, someone you love is gone.

However, his funeral was a roaring success, which is exactly what he would have wanted. That's the great thing about Irish funerals: they're like a big party, the perfect send-off. Although I still miss him every day, I'm glad that we were close and were great friends when he died.

I speak about my dad a lot because I love remembering him. It's only when I've had a drink that I might get upset. I suppose it's because, in a weird way, I blame myself a little for him dying. I pushed him to get the operation out of the way when, maybe, he should have waited a little longer and had more of a life. I also feel I should have been more vocal when he didn't seem right after the operation, because they might have caught his last stroke earlier, but such is life.

When Brian and I first arrived in Australia, only a few months had passed since my dad's death and I was still reeling. I found it difficult to get work and it was hard to have nothing to take my mind off it. When almost six months had gone by with no job, I told Brian that I would have to go home as my money was running out. But, luckily, I landed a stint on *Dancing with the Stars*, which I really enjoyed – though dancing is definitely not my forte. This led to some other TV work, and I did lots of DJing.

Brian and I had a lot of fun when we first got together, though perhaps we partied too much – but isn't that always the way at the start of a relationship? And he was really supportive of me during a difficult time. My family were quite concerned for me because I upped and left the country with someone I had just met, and all the media attention surrounding Brian didn't help the situation. But when they finally met him they understood how much we meant to each other, though they still wanted me to come home.

Brian and I decided to move to the UK in 2014, which I was delighted about. I liked Australia but I really missed my family and wanted to get back to their side of the world. I started working with RTÉ in Ireland again and also did some work in the UK.

Unfortunately, shortly afterwards, Brian and I decided to go our separate ways. I don't want to say too much about the break-up of my marriage because it's in the past and that's where I want to keep it. Brian and I had been struggling as a couple for some time before we announced our split. We had always been friends – that wasn't the problem – but we just couldn't make a relationship work.

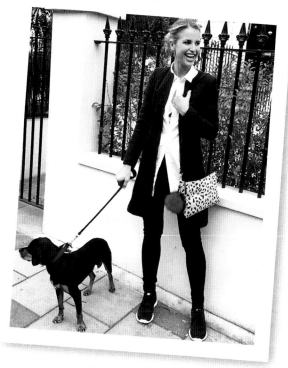

Winston.

The papers were constantly writing about us being back together and, at one point, they weren't totally wrong – it's why everyone thought our split was so amicable – but we were just trying to work it out. It's harder being friends now that we've totally drawn a line under our marriage. I wouldn't want to bad-mouth Brian in my book because there are, of course, two sides to every story and it's not my style to put it all out there. But we are no longer friends and although I am very good friends with my other ex Al I can't imagine I'll ever be friends with Brian again, our lives no longer fit together in any way. I found the whole divorce process very difficult but when I got the signed papers back, I felt such relief and like I had the ability to move on properly from that part of my life.

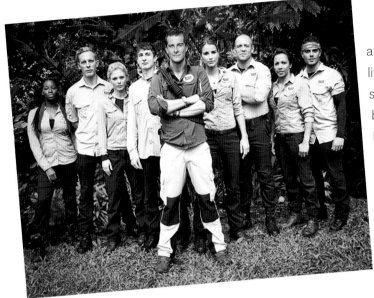

While I was going through a tough time in my personal life, my professional life had started to go really well. I booked my first series in Ireland in 2015, entitled *Vogue's Wild Girls*, which was a follow-up to a previous standalone episode, *Vogue Does Straight As*. This time, I had a three-part series: the first part focused on the American prison system, which saw me meeting the youngest girl on death row; the second was on female fighters; and the final part was on sex, which was a hilarious episode to make – I ended up at a swingers' party!

I also took part in the reality show *Mission Survive* with Bear Grylls in which eight of us spent twelve days in a jungle in Costa Rica. It was really tough and I loved every minute of it. Bear pushed us all and I made a lot of good friends from that show. I ended up winning, which was the icing on the cake and not something I had expected. I wanted to do the show because I was attracted to the challenge of it, but I hadn't realised how much I would be able to push myself. It's nice to be surprised, sometimes, by how much I'm capable of when I put my mind to it – definitely an important lesson I've carried with me ever since.

Then I booked a second series with RTÉ, which aired in 2016, entitled *Vogue Williams – On the Edge*. This time it was a four-part series and covered topics that I've always had an interest in – the transgender community, people who are obsessed with their appearance, drug use and abuse, and the dangers of the internet.

I'd always enjoyed watching documentaries, especially ones that followed people's personal stories and the struggles they faced. Like many people, these were one of the main ways I learned about issues. It was fantastic to be given the chance to make my own documentaries and to explore some of the subjects that really interested me in more depth.

And, while I know I've had a good life and am so lucky with my friends and family, in particular, my parents' separation and my dad's death were really tough for me. These experiences changed me profoundly, making me more aware of what people go through (even people who seem very together and happy on the surface). And I've definitely found myself trying harder to walk in other people's shoes, to better understand them and how I might be able to help in some way.

The series was a success – I am very proud of it – and, at the time of writing, I've been commissioned for another series (which will air during 2017). I adore making documentaries and it's something I hope to keep up for the rest of my life.

In early 2017 I took part in *The Jump*, a ski challenge show on Channel 4 – something I had always wanted to do. I had the best time taking part in the show and made some lifelong friends. Unfortunately, after six weeks of training in Austria I got injured, just days before the live shows began. To say I was devastated is an understatement. I had worked so hard and just like that, I was out without ever experiencing one show.

I had a nasty fall during a training session, and every time I tried to stand up, I just kept falling over because my knee was so painful and unstable. I had no idea what was wrong

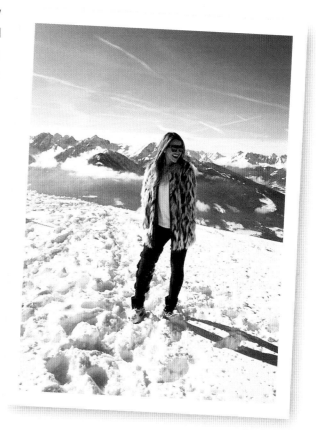

but everyone else in the group had a feeling it might be more serious than I thought. Despite this, I was insistent on getting the ski mobile down the hill even though they wanted me in a stretcher. I also refused the gas because I just thought they were trying to make good TV and that I would be skiing again in the morning! It turned out that I had snapped the ACL (anterior cruciate ligament) in my right knee. I was in a lot of pain, and really disappointed to miss out on the show, but the cast and crew helped me through, and couldn't have done enough for me.

I ended up having an operation on my knee to replace my snapped ACL with some of my hamstring. I struggled with the operation, and was a bit unrealistic about the healing process, booking a job for two days after my surgery thinking I would be fine! It's been a very long road to recovery with endless hours in physio but I've worked really hard at it so I'm almost 100% better. I loved the show so much that I'm trying my very best to be back on form to do it all over again next year.

I also met my boyfriend Spencer on *The Jump*. We became great friends from the moment we met and spent all of our time together in Austria. I suppose it was a strange situation because we were practically living together from day one but I'm really glad it happened that way. He's such an amazing person and it's nice to be in love again. He's one of the most chilled people I know and is always in a good mood. I think his positivity definitely rubs off on me and whenever I'm with him I feel really happy which is a pretty great way to feel with someone. And he's really supportive of everything I do.

I still do a lot of modelling and DJing, travelling back and forth between Ireland and England. I write a weekly newspaper column as well as a weekly blog for *Hello!* magazine. I did have a radio show for a year, which allowed me to showcase my love of music, but I couldn't keep it on, unfortunately, as I got too busy.

A lot of people ask me how I fit all of it in but everything just seems to come together – though I definitely have my days where I feel like I've taken on too much. There are the days when I'm missing out on a big event or family gathering because of my job, but I love what I do so I get over the FOMO quite quickly. My newest trick is to never look more than a week ahead in my diary so I don't stress myself out! I have always enjoyed working and like to give a hundred per cent to everything I do. I am a firm believer that if you work hard enough and focus on what you want to achieve, anything is possible. The harder you work, the luckier you will get. Of course, some people are fortunate enough to have more opportunities than others, so you have to try to make the most of every opportunity that comes your way. And, hopefully, there'll come a time when you'll have the chance to present someone else with an opportunity.

Though I enjoy my job, it's really important to balance hard work with physical and mental health, but it's a difficult thing to get right. I prefer to think of it as a work in progress, and don't give myself a hard time when I could be doing a better job of it.

I'm a big fan of writing things down as a way of making plans and working through what I have going on, especially during stressful periods, so when the opportunity came along to write this book, I jumped at it. As well as the achievement of an ambition, it's been a really therapeutic process and an interesting way for me to examine my approach to everything.

Another part of my approach to combatting stress and anxiety is fitness, which has played a huge role in my life ever since I was a teenager. When I split up with Brian, for example, the gym was a place where I could work out my emotions and clear my head. And keeping fit has been a huge boost to my overall health, as well as something I enjoy. Over the years, I have learned a lot about how to fuel my body properly without ever being on a diet, and what I eat plays an important part in how I feel every day. I love food and believe it's there to be enjoyed. I find it to be a really sociable thing too. Dinner parties with friends are my way to relax and catch up with people I haven't seen in ages. And I love cooking for people.

I don't have the perfect body – who does? – but I've learned that exercise, eating the right food, taking care of my appearance and wearing clothes I feel comfortable in makes me look and feel my best. Everyone can achieve this confidence – it's just about making small changes to your life and knowing what suits you. And spending time on yourself – whether this means going for a walk, having a facial, going for lunch with friends or meditating – is an essential part of everyday life.

Ultimately, with my book, I want everyone to find their confident place and make sure they have fun in the process. If you want that glass of wine, have it – just make more healthy choices the next day. We're all different and that is what makes us great, and I hope that by sharing the tips that help make me feel confident, you will feel confident too.

# Anxiety

Anxiety plays quite a big part in my life, and I'm sure it does in a lot of other people's too. It's very hard to explain where these anxious feelings come from for me, but they often take over when I'm really busy or haven't been sleeping well. Anxiety is a strange thing to explain, especially to someone who doesn't have it – mine can cause sleepless nights, pains in my stomach and an overwhelming sense of worry.

My anxiety started in my early twenties, though I didn't realise it was anxiety at the time – I just thought I was really stressed. I regularly had what is commonly described as 'the fear': an overwhelming sense of everything closing in on me and a constant worry about what might happen in the future.

I began doing a lot of modelling when I was about twenty years old, and it was around that time that the details of my life became more public. One of the things I hadn't considered was that people would be discussing and making judgements about the choices I make and the way I live my life – and I don't think I was really prepared for that. I have learned how to handle it better over the years, but it can still be difficult. I wouldn't say my chosen career is why I have anxiety, but it definitely contributes to it.

When I'm having a bad day, anxiety will be lurking underneath everything while I try my best to get on with things. I think the worst it has ever been was when, in 2016, I went away on a retreat. I was very excited about the trip, but I had a lot going on in my personal life and so wasn't feeling great from the start. I really enjoyed the retreat overall, but I couldn't get my anxiety to go away. It was hanging over me all day and then, at night, it was difficult to sleep because my mind was racing. When I eventually did drop off, I was woken up throughout the night by pains in my stomach and a horrible sense of worry that something terrible was going to happen. It was the first time I had let it get the better of me. After two days, I was really upset and exhausted and knew I had to go home. I felt the need to be somewhere familiar with my friends around me and, though I felt a bit defeated, it was the right thing to do.

Luckily, these bad days aren't a regular occurrence, but when they do happen I feel sick. I struggle to eat anything and I just want to stay inside my house until the feeling goes away.

And bad days can make working difficult because the last thing I want is to be surrounded by people I don't know, having to hide that I feel awful. But, generally, I find that making myself continue with business as usual can help, because there is no choice for me but to put it to the back of my mind. Of course, this won't necessarily work for everyone – we're all different – so it's important to figure out what helps you.

In 2016, my anxiety was quite bad in general. I slept poorly during the night, and I woke up with stomach pains almost every day. Some days I found it hard to get out of bed until they had subsided slightly. I had tried to 'fix' my anxiety myself for quite some time – I don't think there's anything wrong in taking medication when it's needed, but I wanted to exhaust all of my other options first. Unfortunately that hadn't really worked, and at this point, I knew I needed some extra help. So I decided I should see a doctor.

I ended up going on beta-blockers for a few months. They helped to block out everything negative about my anxiety and I was able to continue my day as normal. After a few months on this medication, I felt I could stop taking it, as I was in a better place in my life and felt happier in general. I was glad that I'd made the

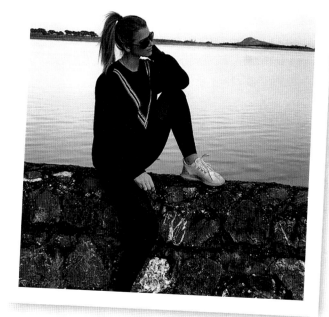

When I'm having a bad day, anxiety will be lurking underneath everything while I try my best to get on with things.

decision to go to the doctor, and the medication definitely helped, but at the moment, thankfully, I'm able to manage my anxiety without it.

When I feel an anxiety attack coming on – usually it starts with stomach pain for me – I try to take ten minutes away from whatever I'm doing and meditate or just take deep breaths. I focus on nothing but trying to calm myself. A trick that was recommended, and really works for me, is this: take deep breaths and imagine you're breathing in a white light. Then, when you exhale, imagine you're blowing out black smoke. It might sound a little odd, but it focuses my mind on the task and makes me feel calmer.

I think it's important to make space in your daily life for mindfulness – time for yourself, when you do absolutely nothing but be in the moment. Meditating is a great way to do this and can be done in loads of different ways. I have a very short attention span and am always thinking of the next thing, so meditating does not come easy to me. I've tried meditating with apps and to music, but I either fall asleep or my brain keeps going a million miles an hour. The best way for me to be mindful is by doing yoga. I don't do it as often as I should, but it's a light workout and it totally calms me down.

Whatever you find works for you, it's important to give yourself at least ten minutes every day where you do absolutely nothing and just totally relax. Being mindful has helped a lot with my anxiety too, so it's why I try to do it every day.

I visit a counsellor when I'm in Ireland and speak to her on the phone regularly too, and I feel that this definitely helps. It's a lot easier to discuss things in your life with an unbiased person who you know isn't judging you or won't get upset the way a family member or friend might at seeing you in pain.

I also spoke with a nutritionist a few years ago who gave me some good general advice on how what I eat and drink can affect my body's response to anxiety. Caffeine is a no-no and alcohol can trigger my anxiety the following day. But I do enjoy socialising and having a drink with friends, so when I'm not feeling the best the next day I live on camomile tea. I also take magnesium twice a day and do my best to eat healthily, and it all helps, if only a little.

But the biggest helper for me is definitely exercise. Everyone knows exercise can lift your mood and this is one reason why it occupies such a pivotal role in my life. It makes you feel good and it makes you look good too – total winner!

I was uncertain whether or not to talk about my anxiety openly in this book. I know that I have a good life – anxiety being just a small part of it – and I don't want to sound like a moaner. But there is a stigma attached to anxiety – and to mental health issues in general. Whenever I have discussed my experiences in interviews, I've received messages from people going through something similar. If I can help in any way to reduce this stigma or to offer comfort to someone, that's a hugely positive thing and I'm happy to do it. Anxiety is not something to be ignored or laughed at, because it is such a real thing for so many people. Perhaps some of the tips I've mentioned above will help anyone reading this who suffers from anxiety, but, if they don't, remember that everyone is different and there is plenty of help out there – you just need to find what works for you.

I think it's important to make space in your daily life – time for yourself.

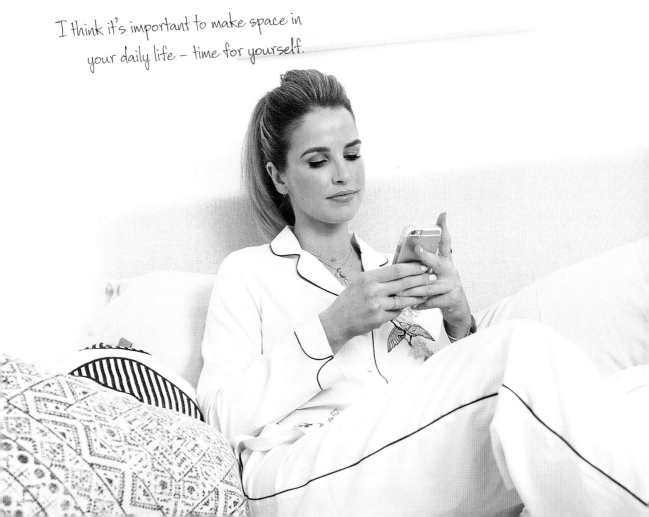

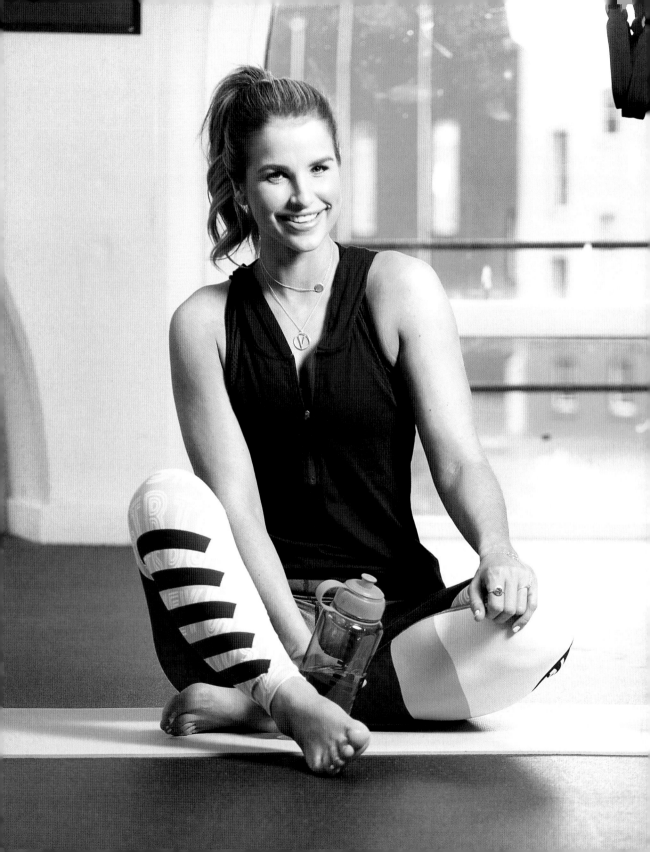

# Fitness

Fitness has become a huge part of my life in the past few years. I loved sports as a child and I have always had a competitive edge to my personality – something my siblings are very aware of! I started going to the gym on a regular basis when I was about eighteen – Ireland doesn't have very dependable weather for sports or exercising outside, and it worked well for me to be able to fit gym visits around my schedule rather than having to plan around a training session or class. But despite this, I have really only recently learned how to train my body properly.

There is a misconception that the longer your workout sessions are, the better you will look – and that is just not true. I have recently halved the length of the workouts I do – I used to do an hour – so I never spend longer than 30 minutes in the gym and I am in the best shape I have ever been in.

I do think it's important to get a schedule together – having no time is not an excuse. It's important to *make* time. This can be really tough – it's so tempting to spend that extra half an hour in bed or to change into pyjamas rather than workout gear in the evenings (believe me, I know!) – but the benefits of dedicating time to fitness are huge. I know that I always feel great after a workout – it gives me energy, clears my mind and usually improves my mood. As mentioned in the previous section, it's an

important part of my self-care when it comes to mental health. And, though I know not everyone finds this, I really enjoy working out – I like to push myself and see my body getting stronger every day.

*I always feel great after a workout – it gives me energy, clears my mind and usually improves my mood.*

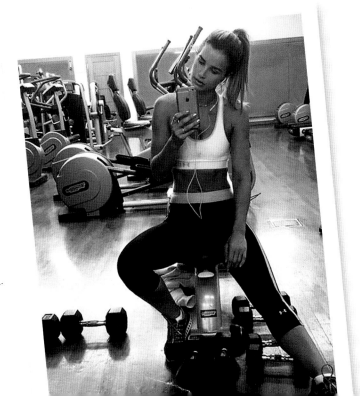

26

It can make a difference to find something you enjoy doing – whether it's a peaceful morning swim, or a brisk stroll during your lunch break, or running with friends in the evenings. I think everyone can find between twenty and thirty minutes a day to improve their fitness. If you are struggling with that, then incorporate getting fit into your daily routine in other ways – do squats while you wait for the kettle to boil; do burpees while your bath is running – just make sure you get it done.

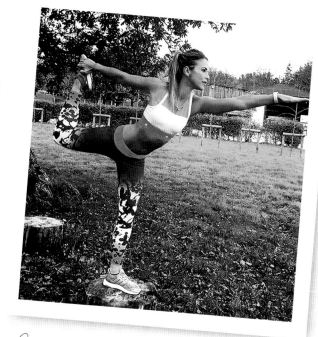

*Everyone can find between twenty and thirty minutes a day to improve their fitness.*

Don't be put off if you don't lose weight through exercise. I have been the same weight for years, but I am more toned now and have lost inches. Remember that muscle weighs more than fat so ditch the scales and go by how your clothes fit instead – and how you feel!

In this section, I have included fitness routines I use on a regular basis for you to try out. I know it can be difficult to fit workouts into your schedule, but use it as your 'me' time. If you really want to start training – whether it's to lose weight, to get healthy or just for fun – these routines are easy and most of them can be done at home.

# For Beginners

It can be quite daunting to start training. Whether you're a size eight or a size twenty-four, the gym can be a scary place. Not knowing how to do certain exercises can be embarrassing, but everyone has to start somewhere and at least you are beginning your fitness journey, so all power to you!

Getting a personal trainer when you are starting out is a great option, but it can be very expensive. Gyms have their own trainers who are there to help you – so if you join a gym, make sure you avail of their advice. Many of them will also help you to develop a workout routine to suit your needs. Going to classes can be helpful too, and less expensive, but try and join one that doesn't have many people in it. If the class size is quite small, the trainer can pay more attention to how you're doing and ensure you're doing the exercises correctly – you can really injure yourself if you do an exercise the wrong way. And don't be afraid to ask for help or advice if you need it! I still go to classes because I love the company. And going with friends can make it fun, although my friend Ashley and I are always separated for being too chatty!

If you feel that the gym is too daunting to begin with, you could start by power walking or jogging and work your way up to it. You can do home workouts like I've included below or take some other routes to getting fit – maybe joining a group that does an activity like running or cycling together; becoming a member of a sports team; buying a workout DVD; or using online resources, such as training videos. I do lots of training videos on my Instagram account so check them out if you're looking for some inspiration!

## Training gear

To say I'm obsessed with training gear is an understatement – it's my favourite present to receive from anyone and I've become a training-gear hoarder! I definitely don't need fifty pairs of leggings, but I have them anyway. I like having nice things to wear to the

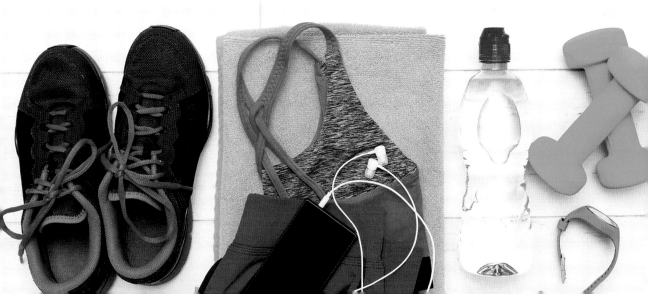

gym because I go so often and it's important to be comfortable when I'm working out. Do make sure your gear ticks both boxes – I learned my lesson from the time I wore some gorgeous new leggings to the gym but had to leave early because they kept falling down.

I like to wear leggings that come up to just below my belly button and are super tight. When it comes to choosing what you wear on your bottom half, just make sure you don't choose tracksuit pants that are too long, as you'll be in danger of tripping up, or too loose, as they'll fall down. I don't have big boobs, so I can wear any sports bra, more or less, but if you are bigger in the bust, you should find one that will give you good support, which is especially important for exercises that involve a lot of movement. Otherwise you'll find working out uncomfortable.

There are so many options out there for gym gear, and pieces don't have to be expensive to be good, so make sure you shop around. I always try on everything before I buy and do a test squat and lunge to make sure they fit properly. Keep how you'll be exercising in mind when you shop – for example, if you'll be outside a lot, you might want lots of light layers as well as clothes that will keep you dry.

Runners (or trainers, as my UK friends would say!) are the most important part of any gym kit – I've had runners in the past that had no support and I've ended up nearly spraining my ankle. There are a lot of brands out there and most of them are good but, again, it's about trying them on and getting a pair suited to your training. I like to do a bit of research online before buying and I ask for advice from the assistant at the shop – they're usually well informed about which shoes work best for the type of exercise you have in mind.

## My top tips for buying workout gear

☆ Make sure you try on everything before you buy – it may look nice but that doesn't always mean it's comfortable.

☆ Get a sports bra that's suited to you and has been fitted properly. You don't want to get a boob in the face on the treadmill!

☆ Always make sure that your leggings are quite high-waisted. If you're squatting and lunging, you don't want your bum coming out to say hi!

☆ Don't spend a fortune. The most expensive gym gear isn't always guaranteed to be the best, and there are lots of budget-friendly options available!

## Music

To me, one of the most important things to have when exercising is good music, as I find it really motivating, especially when it's something new. I love all types of music, but I usually listen to rap (my first love when it comes to music) and grime at the gym. I started out listening to electro music, which would get almost anyone moving! I have a huge music collection and I have lots of mixes from my time presenting my radio show. When I trained for an hour, I made these mixes an hour long so they would last me for one session or class in the gym.

I upload a lot of mixes to my Mixcloud account – mixcloud.com/voguewilliams – so people are free to listen to them. They're best suited to working out (or playing at parties) so check them out if you're ever looking for soundtrack suggestions for your next gym session. And I'm addicted to my sister's Spotify account – she has made some really great playlists of music I wouldn't usually listen to, so when I get bored of my own, I listen to hers. You can find these under her username, Ambi Bambi.

## My current top-five artists for gym-listening

1. Skepta
2. Kano
3. ASAP Rocky
4. Soulwax
5. Futrism

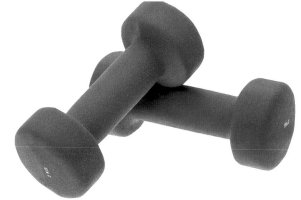

# My Routine

I go to the gym five or six times a week, but three or four sessions is more than enough – I just really enjoy going so I do the extra days. Rest days are very important and it's recommended to take one or two a week. If I wake up in the morning and feel tired and overworked, I take a day off, but I'll still usually go for a walk – this is mainly because Winston, my dog, makes me.

The only time I use cardio equipment at the gym is to do a minute-long sprint on the treadmill. I use weights a lot – this can be body weight with push-ups, free weights and sometimes the machines (though I don't use these very much). As well as sprinting, I do other high-intensity cardio exercises, which can include box jumps, burpees (I despise these, but the benefits are amazing) and mountain climbers.

## Classes

I don't really enjoy training by myself and find it a lot easier when I train with a personal trainer or a friend. But, as this isn't always possible, I often do a class instead – that way I will push myself harder and I won't need to do it alone. Here is a list of the classes I like to do as part of my exercise regime.

1. **Spin:** I love spinning. It's a class you will sweat a lot in, and you have no choice but to push yourself because the teacher will scream at you if you don't! I only spin once a week, as it can really build up your leg muscles and I don't really want to make mine any bigger. Spin classes are for any level of gym-goer: you just work at the level you can on the bike.

2. **Yoga:** Yoga is great for stretching out your body, especially if you have had a tough week at the gym. It's a really calming class and can be quite difficult. And there are lots of different types to try out, such as ashtanga and Bikram (though hot yoga isn't for me – I've tried it a couple of times and find the heat hard to take). I can only ever do yoga as part of a class – I've tried following DVDs at home but I don't do Yoga regularly enough so find it hard to follow the moves. But if you do find yourself able to do it at home, it can be a great way to start the day.

3. **Pilates:** I prefer Pilates to yoga, though I always skip the meditation at the end. I probably shouldn't, but that's something I prefer to do at home in my own house – that way, I feel less self-conscious and have fewer distractions. Sometimes, I do Reformer Pilates, where you use a machine for resistance: it is so much harder than it looks and works all of your muscles. Pilates is fairly similar to yoga, but you use your body weight a little bit more.

4. **High-intensity interval training (HIIT):** HIIT is an absolute killer but one of my favourite classes in the gym. It's like circuit training but a lot more difficult and will definitely make you work up a serious sweat. It involves alternating short periods of intense anaerobic exercise, such as jumping or running, with less intense recovery periods. I love it because I like to feel exhausted after the gym – I sleep much better and feel a fantastic sense of achievement – and a good HIIT class will definitely do this for you.

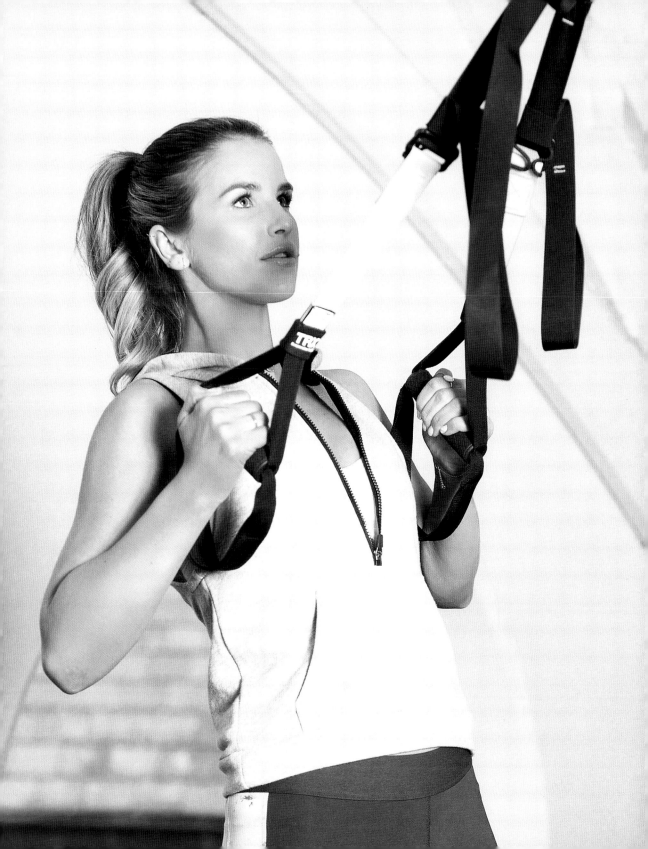

# My Workouts

Here I've compiled a few training routines that can be done easily at home with little to no equipment. Aim to do three or four workouts a week – you can do more if you want, but three is a good place to begin. Start off doing as much as you can and build it up gradually until you can do the whole routine. You'll find that within a couple of weeks of training you'll have mastered most of the exercises and will be feeling so great that it will spur you on to continue. I know that's what happened for me.

## WARMING UP

It's important to warm up at the beginning of a workout, as it reduces muscle soreness the next day as well as your risk of injury, and to cool down at the end to get your body back to a more relaxed heart rate.

For a warm-up, I always do twenty jumping jacks, ten burpees, twenty high knees and repeat this twice. It's enough to get your body warm and ensure you don't pull anything.

## My at-home workout

**Duration:** 4 times takes 35 minutes, 5 times takes 40 minutes
**Exercise type:** cardio and weights
**Benefits:** helps you lose inches
**Frequency:** 3 to 4 times a week

I go to the gym a lot. Sometimes, though, I just don't feel like going or I'm stuck for time but I still want to train. I always try to do a complete body workout, while sometimes also concentrating more on one area like my abs or my tush.

This is my go-to routine that I can do at home or in a park with little equipment –

body weight is enough. I start with Exercise 1, work through to Exercise 7 and repeat this routine four or five times. Then I might add in the ab routines (page 39) or tush routines (page 41) if I have time or want a little extra – so put on a bit of music and get going!

## Exercise 1: jumping squats x 20 reps

1. Stand with your feet shoulder-width apart.
2. Do a regular squat, but as you start to stand up, engage your core and jump up explosively.
3. When you land, lower your body back into the squat position to complete one rep. You should try to land as quietly as possible, which requires control.

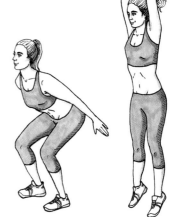

## Exercise 2: press-ups x 12 reps

I alternate between full press-ups (where I'm in plank position) and ones where I'm resting on my knees.

1. Lie on the floor face down and get into plank position, with your arms just outside your shoulders.
2. Lower yourself until your face almost touches the floor.
3. Raise yourself back up to the plank position.

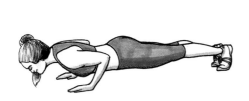
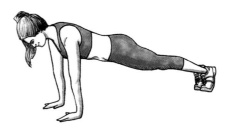

## Exercise 3: jumping lunges x 16 reps

1.    Stand with your feet together, elbows bent 90 degrees, as if you are about to start running.
2.    As you lunge forward, with your right foot, move your left arm up and your right arm down.
3.    From the lunge position, jump straight up as you swing your arms to help you gain height (imagine how you move your arms when you are running). Switch your legs in mid-air, like a scissors, and land in a lunge with your left leg forward and your right arm moving upwards.

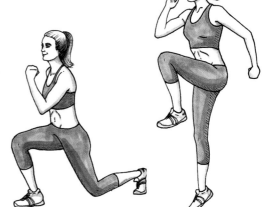

## Exercise 4: tricep dips x 12 reps

I always keep my legs straight to make this exercise a little harder, but you can do it with your knees up.

1.    Sit with your back to a bench or low chair.
2.    Reaching back, place your hands on the bench so your fingers are pointing towards you.
3.    Straighten your arms so that you lift your bum off the floor, keeping your legs straight, only your heels should be touching the floor.
4.    Bend your elbows to lower your bum towards the floor.
5.    Push back up until your elbows are straight.

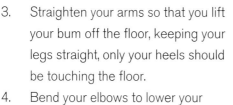

## Exercise 5: wall jumps x 10–15 reps

I tend to do these at a bench in the park, or you can do them at a convenient step at home or in your garden.

1.  Stand with your feet shoulder-width apart, at a comfortable distance from the step or bench.
2.  When you're ready to jump, drop quickly into a quarter squat, then extend your hips, swing your arms, and push your feet through the floor to propel yourself onto the step.
3.  Land lightly and in a squat position.

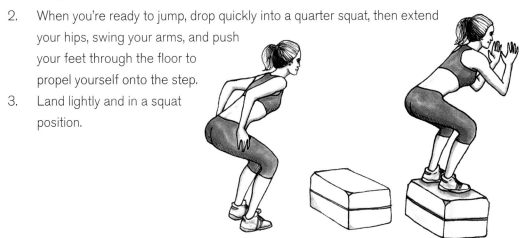

## Exercise 6: bear crawls x 15 metres forwards and backwards

These are so good for your whole body and can be quite exhausting after a while. The title says it all, really: crawl along on all fours!

1.  Start in a plank position, with your knees bent slightly so that there's no dip or arch in your spine.
2.  Going backwards, move your opposite arm and opposite leg at the same time.
3.  Then move forward in the same way.

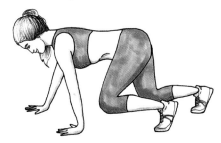

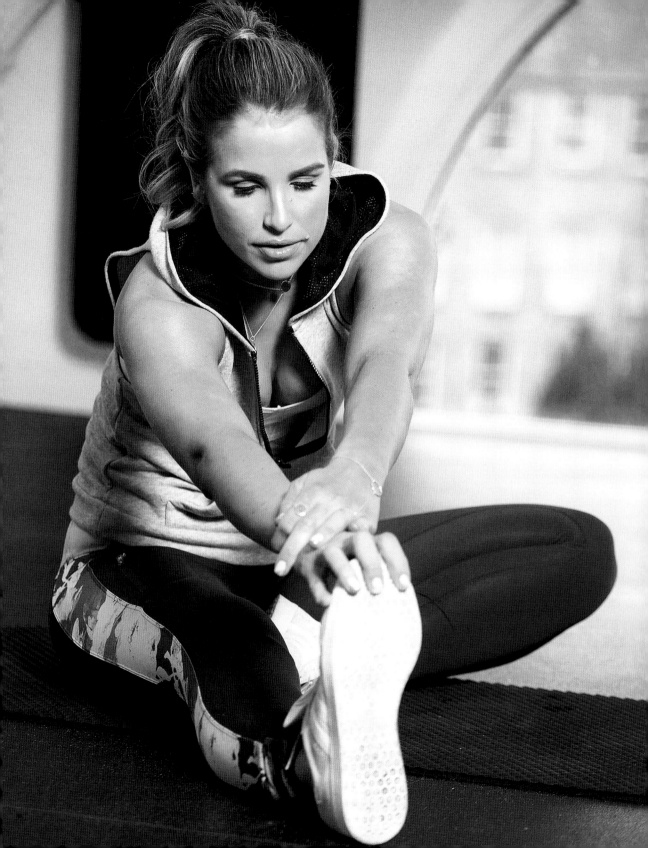

### Exercise 7: burpees x 15 reps

These are one of my least favourite things to do, but they really work! They are high intensity and exercise your entire body.

1. Begin in a standing position.
2. Drop into a squat position with your hands on the ground.
3. Kick your feet back, while keeping your arms extended.
4. Immediately return your feet to the squat position.
5. Jump up from the squat position.

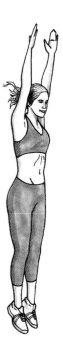

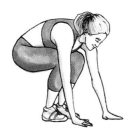
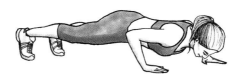

# Ab routines

I was asked recently about the best way to get stronger/more-defined/better abs. We've all heard that abs are made in the kitchen and I somewhat agree with this. I don't think you can have a terrible diet and then train and expect to end up with a six-pack – the two work together. I also don't think that ab exercises alone will give you the stomach definition you want. Weight training involves working your core all of the time, so you are constantly improving your abs without really noticing. I always mix weight training and ab exercises for the best results.

I have a lot of different ab exercises, but below are my top three. I do three rounds of each.

## Bicycle abs

These are great for the sides of your tummy!

1.  Lie flat on the floor with your lower back pressed to the ground, keeping your core muscles contracted.
2.  With your hands gently holding your head, lift your knees to about a 45-degree angle.
3.  Slowly, at first, go through a bicycle-pedalling motion.
4.  Touch your elbows to the opposite knees as you twist back and forth. I try to do forty of these.

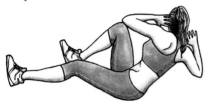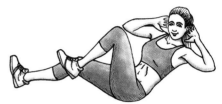

## Ab crunch

These are for your upper stomach and are one of the easiest exercises to see results from.

1.  Lie on your back with your knees bent and feet flat on the floor, hip-width apart.
2.  Place your hands behind your head.
3.  Hold your elbows out to the sides but rounded slightly in.
4.  Lift your head and upper body – make sure that your head, neck and shoulder blades lift off the floor.
5.  Hold for a moment at the top of the movement and then lower slowly back down. I always do twenty of these – you will definitely feel the burn.

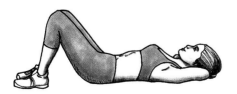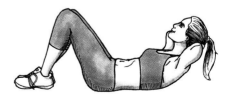

### Leg raises

This one is for your lower stomach muscles, which tend to be the last part to get toned. There are some variations to this exercise, but this is my favourite.

1.  Lie on the ground.
2.  Place your hands under your bum with your palms facing down. Keep your legs as straight as possible. I sometimes use a weight on my legs to make it more difficult.
3.  Slowly raise your legs until they are perpendicular to the floor.
4.  Hold the contraction at the top for one second, then slowly lower your legs to the start position. I do twenty of these.

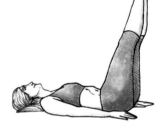

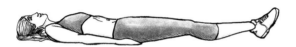

# The Tush

I have become somewhat obsessed with getting the perfect bum! I never used to pay much attention to working out my glutes, but having worked closely with trainers recently, I decided to concentrate more on that part of my body. I bought an exercise band on the internet, which you place around your knees to do these exercises at home. I still do all my gym work but a few times a week I use the band at home to give my bum that extra bit of a workout. And the great thing about the band is that you can take it anywhere: it's so small you could even fit it in your handbag.

Repeat each of the exercises below three times and, voilà, you will be on your way to your dream tush!

## Exercise 1

1. Place the band around your knees and lay back on a bench or on the floor.
2. Bring your heels towards your bum so your knees are bent, but comfortable.
3. Raise your bum off the bench and thrust up and down ten times.

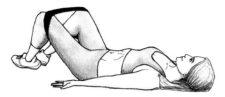 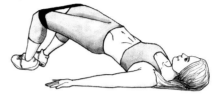

## Exercise 2

With the band still around your knees, and still lying on your back on a bench or the floor with your knees bent, open and close your legs ten times. The resistance of the band will make it hard and you should feel it around your glutes.

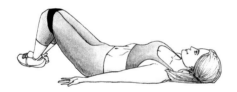 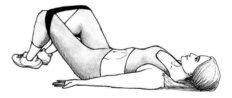

## Exercise 3

1. Stand beside a wall, but sideways on, so your right leg is nearest to the wall (the wall is there so you can use it for balance). Put the band around your knees.
2. Keep your legs straight and raise your left leg outwards, and then lower it again.
3. Repeat ten times.
4. Turn around so your left leg is nearest the wall and repeat the exercise raising your right leg.

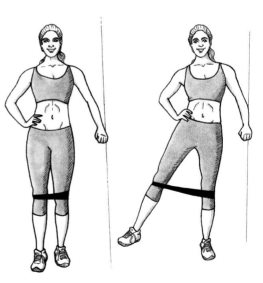

**Exercise 4**

1. Lie on your left-hand side with your knees slightly bent and with the band around your knees.
2. Raise your right leg and lower it again ten times.
3. Turn over so you are lying on your right-hand side and raise your left leg ten times.

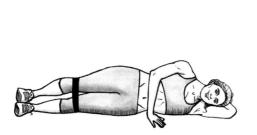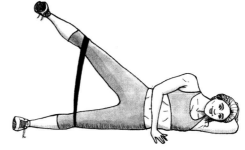

# Trainer Workouts

I could write a million different workouts for you to follow, but I decided to get a few of my favourite trainers to write up some of the workouts we do together in the gym so you will have a good variety of exercises to choose from. I like to switch it up by booking sessions with a number of trusted trainers – that way, I'm being introduced to new ways of working out all the time, and the diverse range of approaches to exercise keeps me interested and on my toes! Below, I've included home workouts from Erica Brennan and Maya Saffronhan, as these complement the workout above, along with a resistance one for the gym. And more workouts for home and the gym are included at the back of the book (pages 250–258), including one from Ollie Frost which I love.

## Trainer workout 1 – Erica Brennan

This is one of the thirty-minute fat-loss home workouts Erica has recommended to me. I work out regularly with her at The Gym Howth, Dublin @thegymhowth. She helped me to get in top shape in the two months before my wedding.

There are five exercises and you should repeat this whole circuit three to five times, depending on how much time you have to spare for the session, with a one-minute rest in between.

**Duration:** 30 minutes
**Frequency:** 3 to 5 times a week
**Benefits:** full-body fat loss
**Equipment needed:** none

## Exercise 1: quarter squats x 25 reps

1. Stand with your feet shoulder-width apart. If your lower body flexibility is poor, put a mat under your heels to elevate them. You need to be able to squat so that your hamstrings and calves touch. This will work all your muscles and use your joints properly.
2. Squat down, pause for 1 second.
3. Lift up halfway, pause for 1 second.
4. Squat down again, pause for 1 second.
5. Lift to standing, squeezing your bum and driving your hips forward.
6. Repeat for 25 repetitions.

## Exercise 2: back extension with walking plank x 15 reps

1. Lie flat on your belly with your arms stretched down by your sides and in the air like aeroplane wings.
2. Take a deep breath.
3. Engaging your abs, exhale and lift your chest off the floor. Keep looking down.
4. Hold and squeeze your bum for 5 seconds.
5. Repeat for 5 reps.
6. Then, place your elbows on the floor under your shoulders, with your hands palms down,  keep your head in line with your spine and keep your legs long on the mat.

7. Tuck your toes under and lift yourself up into a plank (if there was a plank of wood on your back, it would be straight. Don't lift your bum high in the air, look straight ahead.

8. In your plank position, keep your upper body still and move your right foot out to the right (leg straight), tap your toe off the floor and return it back. Do the same with the left foot.

9. Repeat for 5 reps each side.

    --- that's one full set ---

10. Repeat the whole process 5 times.

## Exercise 3: lunge and reach x 30 reps

1. Standing tall with your feet shoulder-width apart, place your hands on your hips.

2. Lunge your right foot forward.

3. Let your chest fall onto your quad.

4. Place your hands flat on the floor either side of your right foot and hold there for one second. Then shoot your foot back into the starting position (this will seriously use your bum).

5. Repeat on your left side and then alternate each leg for thirty reps.

## Exercise 4: push-ups x 15 reps

1. Lie flat on your belly with your hands under your shoulders. Your legs should be straight and your toes tucked under.

2. Exhale and lift your head, chest and belly off the floor. Push the weight into your arms and feet.

3. Slowly return back to the floor and repeat for fifteen reps.

## Exercise 5: burpees x 15 reps

1. Start in a full-body plank (on your hands and feet: knees, hips and chest in the air), toes tucked under.

2. Jump both feet out wide, then jump them back in.
3. Jump your feet back in together so your knees are into your chest.
4. Jump high in the air and clap your hands over your head.
5. Repeat this as fast as you can for fifteen reps.

# Trainer workout 2 – Erica Brennan

**Duration:** 30 minutes
**Frequency:** Three to four times a week
**Benefits:** ABS! ABS! ABS!
**Equipment needed:** None

Repeat this workout three to five times, depending on how much time you have.

## Exercise 1: full sit-ups with twist x 20 reps

1. Lying on your back, arms stretched on the floor behind your head, legs are long on the floor and wide.
2. Breathe in and when you exhale, lift your upper body up off the floor and with your right hand reach down to your left foot (giving your torso a little twist).
3. Slowly go back to the floor and repeat on your other side.
4. Repeat for 20 reps (10 each side).

## Exercise 2: mountain climbers x 60 reps

1. Start in a full-body plank (on your hands and feet – knees, hips and chest in the air), toes tucked under.
2. Bring your right knee in so it is under your chest.
3. Explosively, change the position of your legs so your right leg is extended back and your left knee is brought in to your chest.
4. Repeat this as fast as you can.

### Exercise 3: reverse curls x 40 reps

1. Lie flat on your back with your legs straight up in the air and your hands on the floor either side of you.
2. Lift your hips half an inch off the floor. There should be no momentum – don't swing your legs.
3. Return your hips back down and repeat 40 times.

   (Please note: the lower your lift, the harder it is.)

### Exercise 4: single-side jack knifes

1. Lying on your back, arms stretched on the floor over your head (hugging your ears), legs are long on the floor and are together.
2. Breathe in and when you exhale, lift your legs up off the floor straight up to the ceiling. Simultaneously, lift your upper body up off the floor and reach your clasped hands around your legs to your right-hand side.
3. Bring your whole body back to the floor and repeat on your other side.
4. Repeat for 20 reps (10 each side).

### Exercise 5: half burpees x 20 reps

1. Start in a full-body plank (on your hands and feet – knees, hips and chest in the air), toes tucked under.
2. Jump both feet back in together so your knees are into your chest.
3. Jump them straight back out again.
4. Repeat as fast as you can for 20 reps.

### Exercise 6: plank x 1 min

1. Place your elbows on the floor under your shoulders, with your hands palms down, keep your head in line with your spine and keep your legs long on the mat.

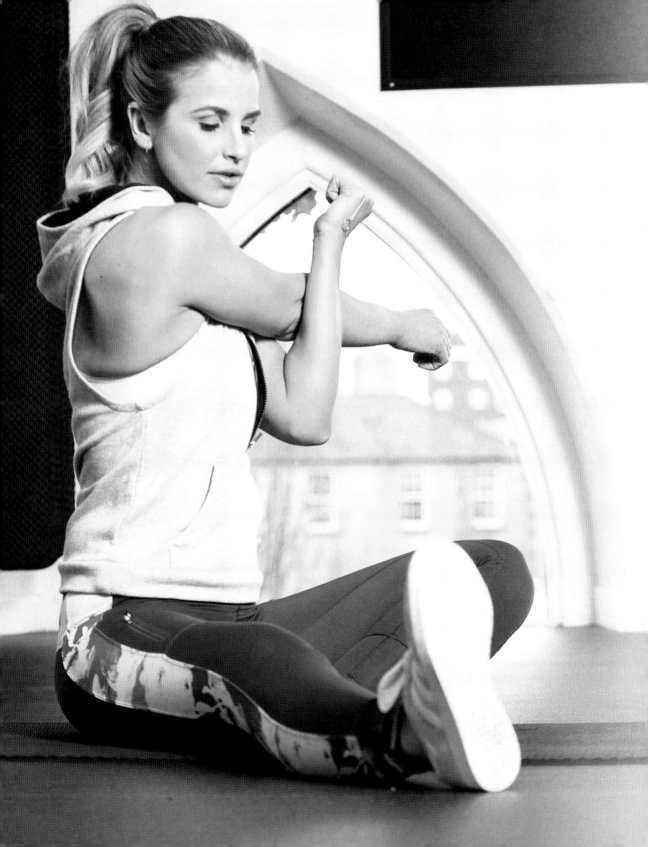

2.    Tuck your toes under and lift yourself up into a plank (don't lift your bum high in the air, look straight ahead).

3.    Stay there!

# Trainer workout 3 – Maya Saffron

Maya Saffron (⊙ @mayasaffronhan), based at Virgin Active in London, is a female-only personal trainer, which means she tailors her approach to educating women about fitness, as well as empowering them and inspiring them to be fitter, stronger and happier. She hates seeing women come into the gym and go to the treadmill because they feel like that's all they can/should be doing. She loves seeing women exploring all aspects of the gym with all of its equipment. From TRX squat jumps to pull-ups on the squat rack. I can definitely attest to this – she always does her best to make me feel comfortable in my own skin, as well as giving me great tips on nutrition. Here's an example of one of her cardio workouts.

**Duration:** 40 minutes
**Frequency:** 3 to 4 times a week
**Benefits:** cardio
**Equipment needed:** None

## Exercise 1: backward bear crawls x 10 reps

1.    Get into a plank position, but bend your knees slightly and make sure there's no dip or arch in your spine.

2.    Going backwards, move your opposite arm and opposite leg at the same time.

## Exercise 2: gorillas x 15 reps

1.    Sticking with the animal theme! Crouch onto all fours, with your hands in front of you, and slightly bend your knees.

2. Jump your feet forward to the right of your body, so that they are parallel with your hands.
3. Lift your hands off the floor and move them further forward.
4. Jump again, and keep going, remembering to lift your hands up and move them forward as soon as your feet land.

## Exercise 3: tombstones x 15 reps

1. Jump up with your arms straight above your head and legs straight.
2. Lie back onto the floor, with your hands stretched above your head and your feet straight and toes pointed.
3. Get back up onto your feet and jump up again.

## Exercise 4: body drops x 15 reps

1. This exercise is just a burpee but instead of jumping your legs behind you and then jumping straight back up again, you drop your body to the floor in between. Start with a jump.
2. Lower your body so your hands are on the floor and jump your feet back (like a burpee) until you are in the plank position.
3. Lower your body to the floor in a controlled manner.
4. Push yourself back up to the plank position.
5. Jump to your feet.

# Trainer workout 4 – Maya Saffron

Before I became properly educated about exercise, I would always worry that exercises with weights would make me too muscly looking or bulky. But I know now that lifting weights correctly is one of the fastest ways to burn fat and sculpt your body.

This is a workout to do in the gym, as you will need to use some of the equipment there. There are three circuits to this workout. Do each exercise with a light weight twelve times, then increase the weight and do each exercise ten times, then, finally, use a heavier weight but do each exercise just eight times.

## Exercise 1: goblet squats

1. Hold a kettle bell at your chest, with your back straight and feet a little further than shoulder-width apart. Your toes should be pointed slightly outward.
2. Squat down with your hips moving back, keeping your back straight. Breathe in as you squat.
3. Stand up and return to the starting position. Exhale as you stand up.

## Exercise 2: dumb-bell flyes

1. Lie on a bench with your feet planted firmly on the floor, holding a dumb-bell in each hand.
2. Lift the dumb-bells so they are straight above your chest. You should have a slight bend in your elbow.
3. Lower your arms laterally (outwards) to the side until the dumb-bells are just lower than the bench.
4. Pull your arms back up until the dumb-bells are above your chest. If you feel that it is more effective to add an incline to the bench, do so.

## Exercise 3: military press bar/dumb-bell

Use a bar or a dumb-bell, depending on how strong you feel. Always ask for advice at the gym before lifting weights. The last thing you want is to sustain an injury and be unable to train when you want to.

1. Stand with your back straight and feet shoulder-width apart, have a slight bend in the knees and bring the bar/dumb-bell to your collar bone.
2. Push the bar/dumb-bell up above your head until your arms are straight.
3. Lower and repeat. Start with a very light weight as this exercise will fatigue you at a

faster rate than upper body exercises as it focuses on your shoulder muscles which have a lower supply of oxygen than elsewhere in the body, meaning that they get more tired faster.

## Exercise 4: face pulls

1. Using the pulley machine in the gym, attach the rope equipment to the top of the pulley.
2. With your back straight and a slight bend in your knees, pull the rope towards your face, bend your elbows and separate your arms so your hands go either side of your head. Your shoulder blades should squeeze together.

## Exercise 5: straight-leg deadlifts with bar/dumb-bells

Use a bar or a dumb-bell, depending on how strong you feel.

1. Stand straight with your feet about shoulder-width apart, holding the bar/dumb-bells in front of you, resting on your thighs.
2. Squeeze your shoulder blades together as you bend your knees slightly and push your hips back. Lower the bars or dumb-bells towards the floor, but without touching it (ensuring to keep your shoulder blades squeezed together tightly).
3. Bend your knees until you feel the stretch in the backs of your legs.
4. Stand up straight and squeeze your bum.

So, lots of routines here for you to try and use as a guide to your training regime. Depending on how often you want to train, you can use a different routine each day. I don't use the same routine two days in a row, as I get bored and it's good to alternate the muscles you train from day to day.

Some of the workouts are longer than others – I would save the longer ones for when you have a little bit more time or are full of energy: they are great for weekends.

## COOLING DOWN

It's easy to be lazy about stretching at the end of a workout – it's something I'm very guilty of at times – but it's so, so important! It does take an extra five minutes but it feels so nice to stretch your muscles out after a tough workout. And it will make you feel less sore the next day. I sometimes use a foam roller if a specific part of my body is sore – usually my legs, so I roll them out quite a bit.

# Rest Days

Rest days are just as important as any time spent at the gym. You can't push your muscles non-stop. Working out, especially resistance or weight training, breaks your body tissues down, and rest days allow your muscles, nerves, bones and connective tissue time to rebuild.

Because I train so regularly, I usually only have one rest day a week – this is probably not enough, but exercise really helps keep my anxiety at bay. I always make sure to take this one day off every week to rest my muscles and, on another day, I will take it slightly easier in the gym.

I have an old injury which still causes me problems. I fractured two vertebrae

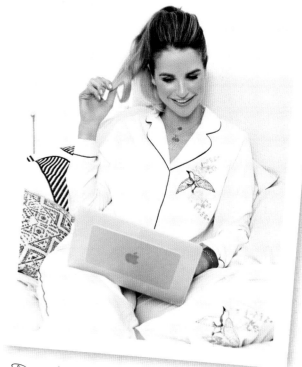

*Rest days allow your muscles, nerves, bones and connective tissue time to rebuild.*

in my back in my early twenties and it still niggles at me, but it can be managed. Strangely, the back injury really affects my knee, which is known as 'referred pain'. And if I haven't been to the chiropractor in a long time, my knee will start to give out. I also find it difficult to find a comfortable way to sit when it's bothering me and that's when I know I need my back sorted. It's very important to be careful of injury. I found out a few years ago from my chiropractor that I have three fractured vertebrae at the bottom of my spine as well as two old fractures on my tail bone. I don't even remember injuring my back but I always felt uncomfortable when I sat or did certain exercises so I avoided them. Now that I know about my injury I can do things to strengthen my back, which really helps with it as well as visits to my chiropractor. Never ignore any type of pain you feel in your body and don't try to train through it because it will only make it worse. Any time I feel strain in my knee following a gym session, I will always ice or strap up the knee and that helps too.

My best advice is to listen to your body – you will know if you've been going at it too hard. And if you do find that you're feeling a bit too sore for training, but you're still keen to do some exercise, you could try something a bit gentler, which will put your muscles through less strain, such as swimming.

## My top tips for staying in shape

☆ **Make a plan:** Being organised is the best way to stay in shape – I've put this first because it's the most important tip. Always make time for training and decide in advance what routine you want to do so you have the necessary equipment ready. If you're doing a gym session in the morning, pack your bag the night before so it's not something you have to think about in the early hours when you're barely awake!

☆ **Push yourself:** I always get asked how I have the motivation to go to the gym and many people say they can't motivate themselves. The thing is, you are the only person who can motivate yourself. You make your own decisions, and if fitness is important to you, you need to make the time for it. I do see staying fit as part of my job, so I make sure training time is always included in my schedule, just like any appointment or meeting. Make it an unmissable part of your day and it will become a habit after three weeks. And because you have made that time in your busy schedule, make sure you give your training session a hundred per cent so it's really worthwhile.

☆ **Sleep:** You always make better decisions when you've had a good night's sleep. A good night's rest makes you feel more energised for your workout session — and much more likely to go in the first place — and, in turn, a training session where you really push yourself will make you sleep so much more soundly.

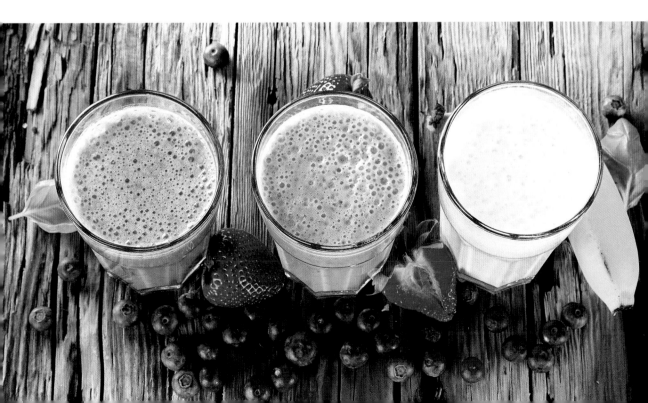

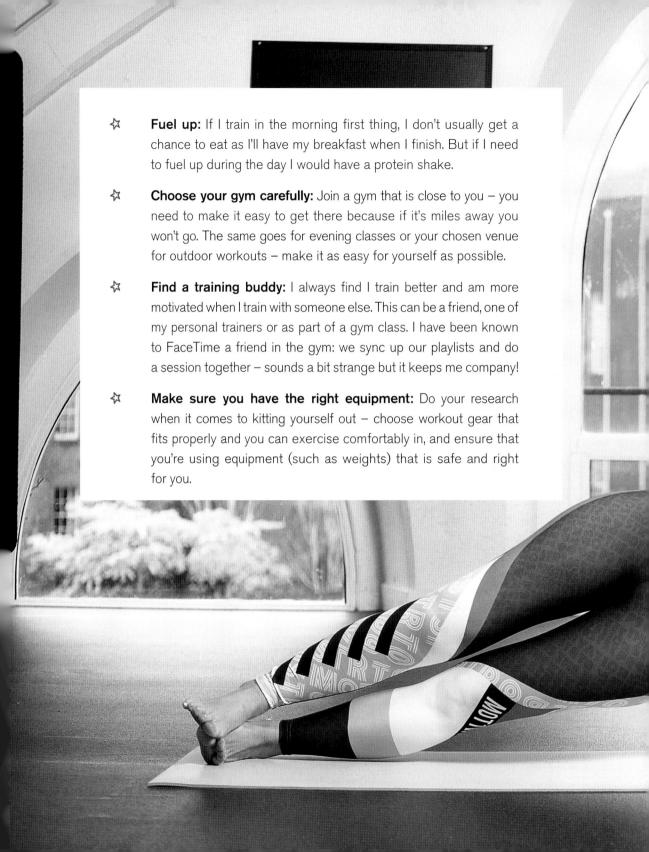

☆ **Fuel up:** If I train in the morning first thing, I don't usually get a chance to eat as I'll have my breakfast when I finish. But if I need to fuel up during the day I would have a protein shake.

☆ **Choose your gym carefully:** Join a gym that is close to you – you need to make it easy to get there because if it's miles away you won't go. The same goes for evening classes or your chosen venue for outdoor workouts – make it as easy for yourself as possible.

☆ **Find a training buddy:** I always find I train better and am more motivated when I train with someone else. This can be a friend, one of my personal trainers or as part of a gym class. I have been known to FaceTime a friend in the gym: we sync up our playlists and do a session together – sounds a bit strange but it keeps me company!

☆ **Make sure you have the right equipment:** Do your research when it comes to kitting yourself out – choose workout gear that fits properly and you can exercise comfortably in, and ensure that you're using equipment (such as weights) that is safe and right for you.

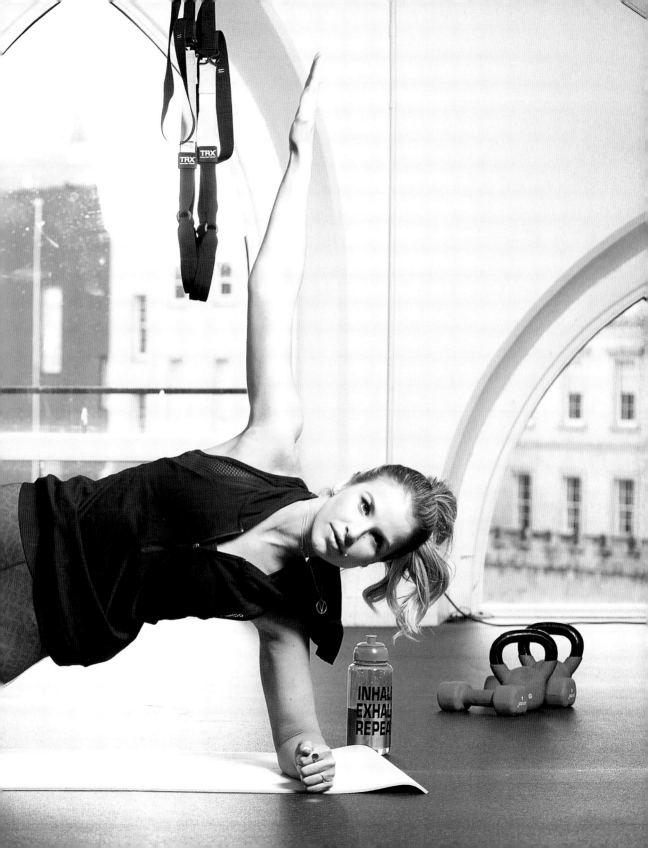

★ **Consider hangover training:** This used to be my idea of hell but recently I have started training when I'm hungover. This obviously depends on the severity – I can only go if I'm just a little hungover. Previously, I used to keep my PJs on and lounge on the couch all day with a big multi-pack of crisps for company. It didn't help the hangover a lot – I just saw it as something I had to ride out. But then I decided to try going to the gym and it made such a difference, leaving me much more clear-headed and energetic. You don't need to spend ages in there but if you can handle going in the first place, you'll end up doing your whole routine and I promise you'll feel much better after.

★ **Rest days:** Remember the importance of a rest day, so you're not pushing your body too hard. And sometimes, when it comes to exercise, life can get in the way, no matter how carefully you're scheduling your workouts. If this happens and you miss a couple of sessions, don't beat yourself up about it. Just do your best to get back to your routine as quickly as possible and re-establish the habit so you can keep building on the hard work you've put in so far.

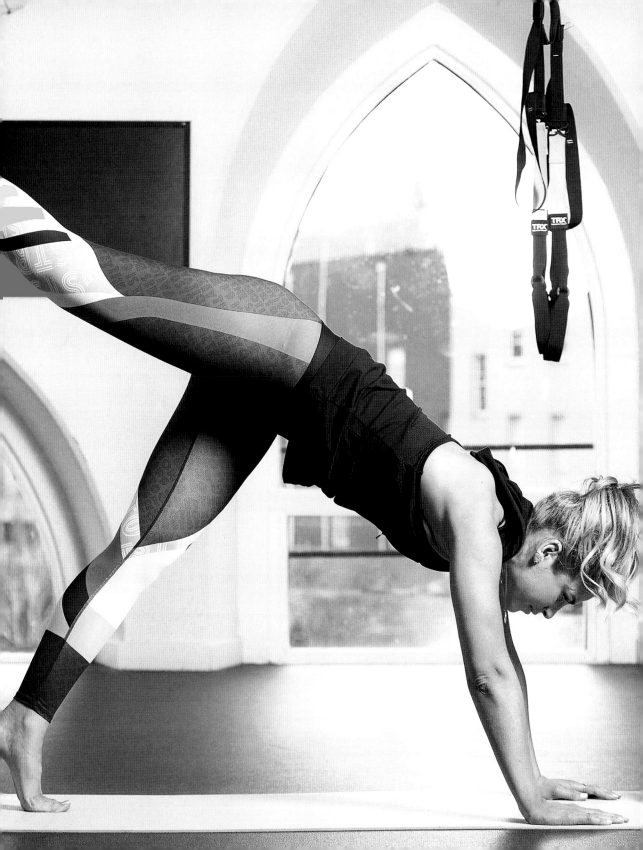

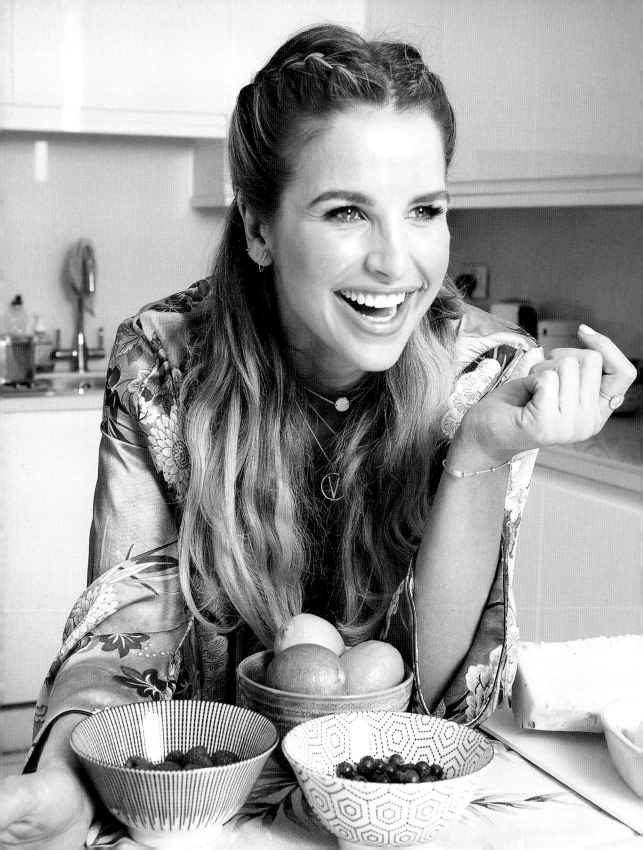

# Food,
# Your Way

My most hated word is 'diet' – I think it sounds scary and impossible. Being on a life-long diet is just not sustainable, and it's not much fun either.

As soon as you forbid yourself anything, you end up wanting it more, and this is especially true when it comes to food. I have tried the odd diet or juice cleanse and, yes, I lost weight on both, but I put it straight back on as soon as I started to eat 'normally' again. Also, who wants to drink cold juice for five days straight? My juice cleanse made me miserable – all I thought about was food!

Personally, I think dieting is a sure-fire way to kill your confidence. When I've tried it in the past, it made me feel horrible and made me hate my body, which is an awful thing. I found it gave me obsessive thought patterns – I spent all my time thinking about what I wanted to eat, what I should be eating and how much I wanted my body to change. And this kind of thinking was not good for me at all. When I talked about it with friends, I found they had the same experience. More often than not, a person on an extreme diet ends up breaking it in a fashion that's just as extreme – and that can leave you feeling even worse. I feel most confident when I've had a great week of healthy eating and training. And I never allow myself to feel hungry – if my body is telling me I need food, I make sure to listen – so my mood is never negatively affected by my eating habits. As you can tell from what you've read so far, exercise is a really big part of my life – and eating right means that my body is fuelled up for a good training session.

The only way to maintain your weight – or lose weight – is through healthy eating and exercise. And food is more important than training when you are trying to get in shape, so it's good to get it right. If you have difficulty sticking to a healthy diet, my advice is plan, plan and do more planning. And do your best to eat as balanced a diet as possible on weekdays and then let yourself go all out one day at the weekend.

It's actually surprising how much you can eat if you consume the right foods – and, remember, fat is not a bad word: good fats are essential in your diet. Eating healthily will have a positive effect on your body, your skin and your hair, and your energy levels will go up.

I've made a big effort to make my own eating habits as simple and delicious and healthy as possible with the busy life I lead, so I've decided to include my favourite meals, snacks and shakes here.

# How I Eat

I am often asked about my diet and people are generally surprised that I eat as much as I do, but everything I eat during the week is healthy.

Now, saying that, if I go out to a restaurant midweek or to a party, I order what I want, which is not always the healthy option – I just eat better the next day. If you are lucky enough to eat out more than once a week, you'd be better off sticking to the healthy options.

## Breakfast

Generally, I wake up around 7 a.m. every day, super excited for breakfast. Breakfast, to me, is the most important meal of the day. I know a lot of people don't like eating as soon as they get up, but you need to so that your metabolism gets a kick start. As soon as I wake up, I'm starving, so my breakfast is always quite big. I usually eat two small pieces of wholegrain toast or brown bread, with half an avocado and two boiled or poached eggs on top. I tend to smother this in

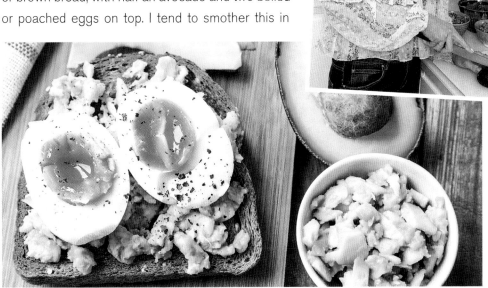

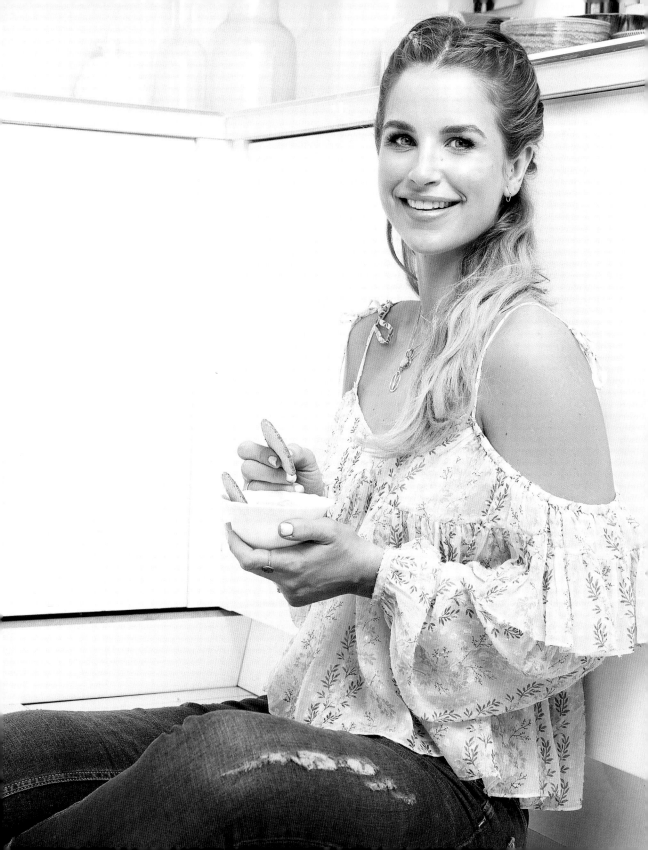

ketchup – I'm working on reducing that because it's full of sugar (but so delicious – I eat it with everything). I don't drink fruit juice because of its high sugar content and it contains extra calories that I don't need, so I have a glass of water and a cup of tea instead.

If you really can't eat something big in the morning, make a healthy shake or have some nuts and fruit. Of course, fruit is full of natural goodness, vitamins and nutrients but I try not to overload on it because of its high levels of sugar – I normally stick to berries or a banana. Everything in moderation.

## Elevenses

My stomach starts talking to me a couple of hours after breakfast so I always have a protein shake or a green juice as a mid-morning snack to keep it happy. It can be so tempting to have a cup of tea and a biscuit instead, but think about how many nutrients you can pack into a shake or juice, and how good that will leave you feeling. I have included a few recipes for these on pages 78–81.

## Lunch

Lunch, for me, is usually eaten on the go, and I'll have a salad box that I have made myself. As with an exercise routine, preparation is key. I set time aside in the mornings to prepare my lunch, making sure that it's as balanced a meal as possible. I find healthy eating is so much easier when you don't have to think too much about what to eat next – I just check my lunchbox to see what's there! Bulgur is my go-to ingredient for lunches (see page 88), and I

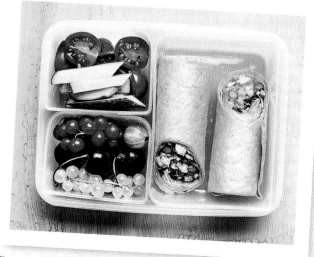

I set time aside in the mornings to prepare my lunch, making sure that it's as balanced a meal as possible.

65

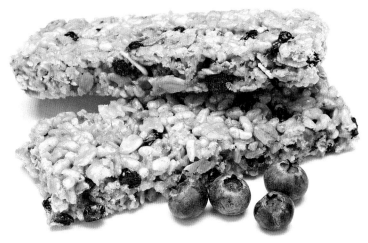

*I make great snack bars in bulk, which I freeze and take them out as I need them.*

make sure to include as much variety as possible when it comes to vegetables. The more colourful the salad, the more nutrients I'm getting. If I have to get lunch when I'm out, I will go for a wrap, salad or soup.

## Afternoon snack

I am always hungry again at around 4 p.m. Snacking is an important part of a healthy diet, though extreme diets often make it sound like a bad thing. For me, it's essential. When my body sugar dips too low, I get tired and cranky – and feeling hungry means it's harder to get things done! This time of day is when my hummus addiction comes into its own. I usually eat hummus and three oat cakes. I also make great snack bars in bulk, which I freeze and take them out as I need them. I've included the recipe for these on page 119.

## Dinner

I never like having to think about dinner when I get home from a long day at work, so I always put aside a few hours a week to cook big portions of food, which I can then freeze for the week (or two) ahead. And it leaves me free to spend time in the evenings doing other things – training, catching up on my favourite TV shows, seeing my friends – instead of slaving over the cooker!

For me, this evening meal is usually chilli (page 96) or a green curry (page 92), with a small portion of brown rice or green veg. I sometimes have fish or steak with vegetables if I have the time to make something from scratch, but, more often than not, I'm too lazy to do that!

## Dessert

I think we all feel unnecessarily hungry after dinner, but for me it's often out of boredom or my sweet tooth kicking in. I have tried treating myself to dark chocolate, but whoever told me I'd want to stop at two squares was a liar – the whole bar ends up disappearing once I start! So for dessert, I love having Greek yoghurt with berries and mixed nuts and a drizzle of agave syrup on top – it satisfies my craving for something sweet, but is a much healthier option than a huge bar of chocolate!

## Blowout days

At the weekend, I usually have one blowout day when I eat anything I want! On a day like this I cook myself a fry shortly after waking up. I always grill everything (except the egg), which is the healthier option, but it's mainly a taste preference for me.

For dinner, I will get a takeaway – either pizza, something from the chipper or a Chinese. And I always like to go to the shop and buy a bag of rubbish – crisps, chocolate, jellies and Capri-Suns.

It's really important to have a cheat day, so that you can have all the stuff you've been craving – and it does make it easier to stick to eating more healthily for the rest of the week. But usually by the time I've finished my blowout cheat day, I am so over unhealthy food that it makes it easier to go back to my healthy eating routine and I don't feel like I've missed out on anything. Of course, you don't need to cheat on every meal – that's

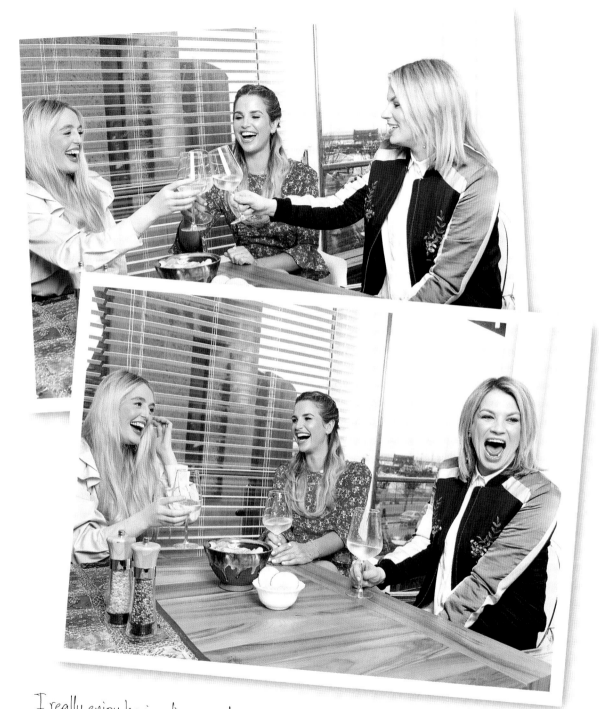

I really enjoy having dinner and a few drinks at home.

just my approach and might be a little extreme for some people. Another option would be to allow yourself a little treat in the evenings, as part of your healthy diet.

Sometimes, my cheat days coincide with a hangover – they're the absolute pits, aren't they? It's the twenty-first century – by now they really should have invented a drink that doesn't give you a hangover! I'm not a huge drinker, but I do like to go out once a week, and because my body isn't used to the alcohol, it affects me quicker during the evening and more forcefully the next day. But I never really consider the thumping headache that will follow when I'm ordering a cocktail! And I have learned some tricks that help me with hangovers, which I'll cover on page 139.

## Dinner parties

I love nothing more than a good dinner party. I really enjoy having dinner and a few drinks with friends in my house or one of theirs. It's a cheap, fun way to socialise, as I'm not a huge fan of going to nightclubs (unless I'm working). Healthy options at a dinner party might sound like a bit of a buzzkill, but you can create a healthy, tasty, Instagram-worthy meal without too much fuss. And then treat yourself and your pals to a nice dessert and a good glass (or two!) of wine.

My mom and Neil live in Spain most of the time and we go to visit them a couple of times a year. While we're there, Mom does the most amazing barbecue, with loads of lovely salads, which I copy when I'm at home – even when it's not sunny or warm, which is usually the case in Ireland and England. I've included some of these recipes further on because they are fairly stress-free and can make hosting a dinner party much easier. Most of the prep is done before anyone arrives, so it gives you more time with your guests.

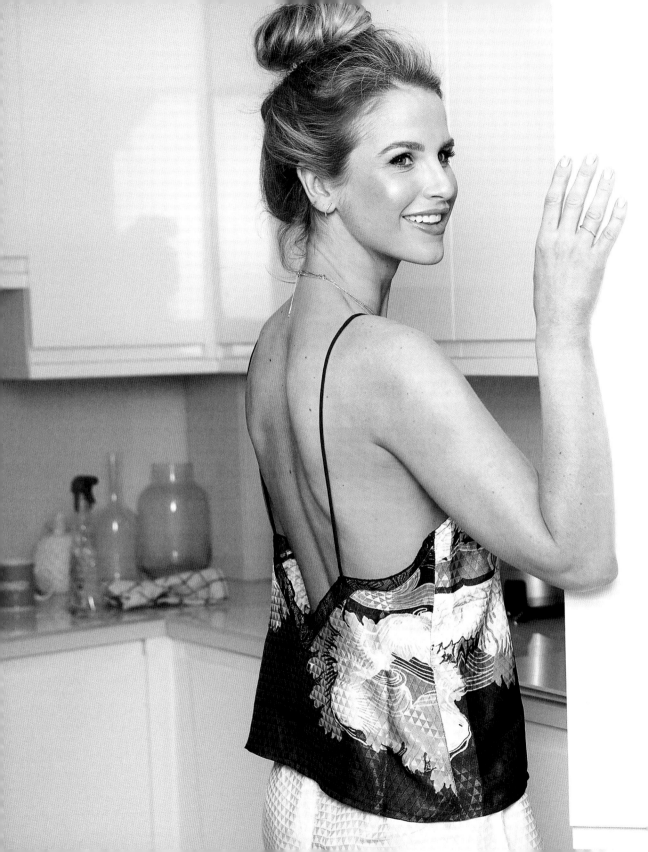

# Recipes

I always enjoy cooking when I have the time. I try to keep it quick and simple – and cook in bulk so I can freeze portions for the coming week. It's the only way to make sure you keep on track with eating healthy home-cooked nutritious food. We all come in from work really tired and the last thing we want to do is cook, which then usually leads to getting a takeaway, but if you prepare at the start of the week, you won't get sucked into taking the unhealthy option.

I've compiled here my favourite healthy recipes for single servings or bigger batches if I'm having people over or if I want to freeze portions. Some of these are from my mom, some are ones I've adapted myself and some are from Dr Tara Coletta, a nutritionist who cooks amazing food that's healthy and delicious. She has worked in the nutrition and fitness field for over fifteen years and has a BKin in Exercise Physiology, an MS in Exercise Science and a PhD in Nutritional Biochemistry and Metabolism. Her objective is to help people find a happy, healthy balance in their life, free of fads and gimmicks. I love Tara's recipes – I find them easy to make and a great source of new ideas! Her recipes are marked with an asterisk.

# BREAKFAST

## Banana pancakes

I eat these for breakfast occasionally because they are so delicious. You can also add flavoured protein powder if you want a different taste, but they are just as nice the way they are!

2 bananas
2 eggs

**To serve**
Fruit – I like to use strawberries, raspberries and/or blueberries
Greek yoghurt agave syrup

1. Mash the bananas in a bowl.
2. Beat the eggs, add to the bananas and mix together. The mixture should have a lumpy texture but you can always put it in a blender to make it smooth if you prefer.
3. Fry on each side in a pan for a couple of minutes and they're ready to go.
4. Pop the fruit, a little Greek yoghurt and some agave syrup on top. Of course, you can add whatever you like to serve, but these are my favourites.

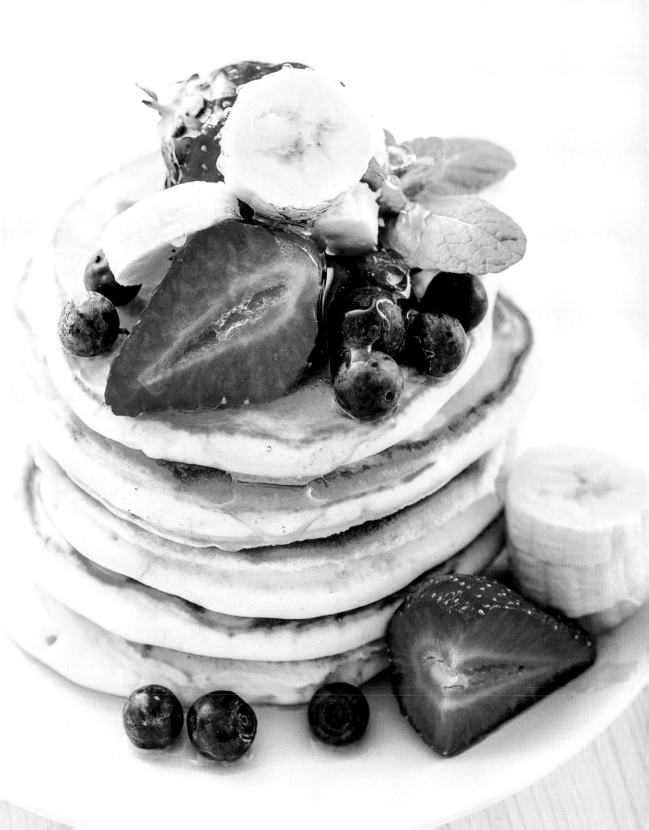

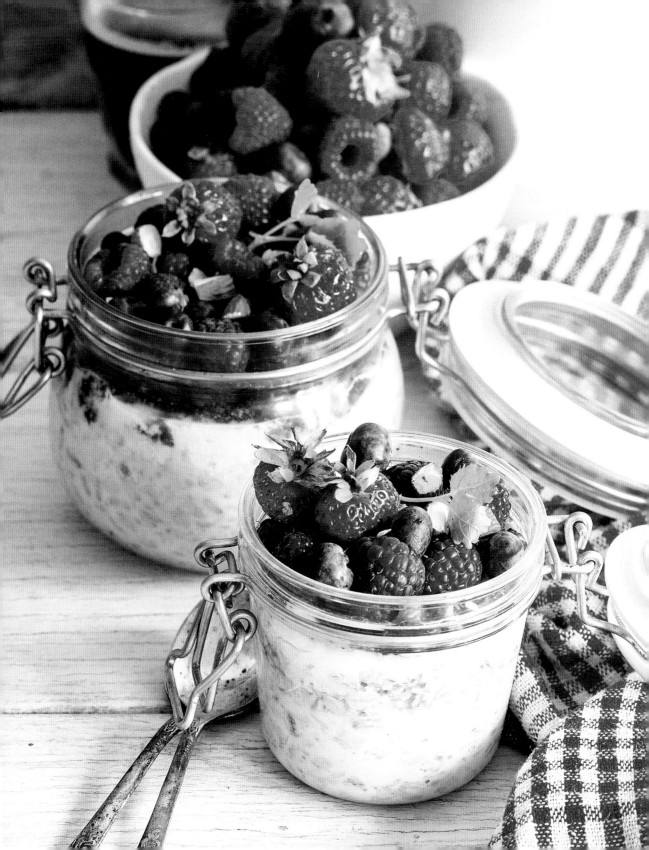

# Bircher muesli

This is one of my favourite breakfasts to have in the summer. It's very easy to make and can be eaten over a few days.

There are many different ways to make it, and you can really mess around with the recipe, substituting fruits and nuts that you prefer. You can also double or triple the portions given, depending on how much you want to have. When I have friends over for breakfast, I always have some of this ready to go – everyone loves it! If you are feeling super healthy you can add a spoon of matcha tea powder, which is so good for you.

½ cup rolled oats
1 tbsp desiccated coconut or chia seeds
handful toasted hazelnuts
handful chopped almonds
raspberries (or any fruit you like – I sometimes add in some blueberries too)
240ml unsweetened almond milk (I switch this up with coconut milk too)
1 tsp agave syrup
pinch of cinnamon
splash of apple juice
1 grated apple

Mix all the ingredients together and leave the mix in the fridge overnight – easy-peasy. You can add more almond milk in the morning just before you start eating.

# Baked avocado

This is so delicious. I cook it if I am having friends over for brunch because it takes minimal effort when everyone arrives. I never like being stuck in the kitchen when I have people over. During the week, I would have a pared-back version without the chorizo, maybe, and use ingredients for one.

3 avocados
6 eggs
half a chorizo sausage
salt and pepper

1.  Cover a baking tray with greaseproof paper and set to one side.
    Preheat the oven to 200°C.
2.  Halve and stone the avocados. If the stone is small, scoop
    out a small bit of avocado so the egg can fit in easily.
3.  Crack one egg into each half of avocado.
4.  Chop the chorizo into small cubes and sprinkle on top.
5.  Season with salt and pepper.
6.  Place the avocados on the baking tray and cook for about 15 minutes.

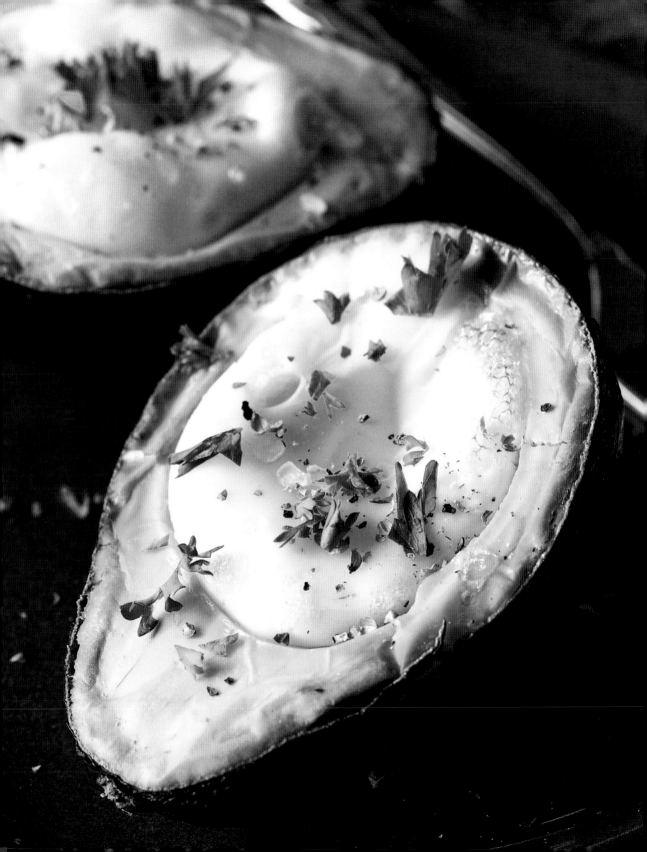

# Green juice

I drink green juices quite a bit because I don't always eat as many vegetables as I should and this is a quick and easy way of getting them into my diet. I've tried so many green juices – some are nice but some taste like mud! I make my own at home as often as I can, as I think they taste nicer and are much fresher. The good thing about a green juice is that you can change the ingredients so it doesn't have to taste the same every time.

1 apple
¼ pineapple
½ avocado
handful of kale
handful of spinach
240ml coconut water

1.  Remove the core of the apple, and the skin of the pineapple and avocado. Stone the avocado. Wash your kale and spinach.
2.  Chop everything into small chunks.
3.  Throw all of it into a blender with the coconut water and blitz until smooth.

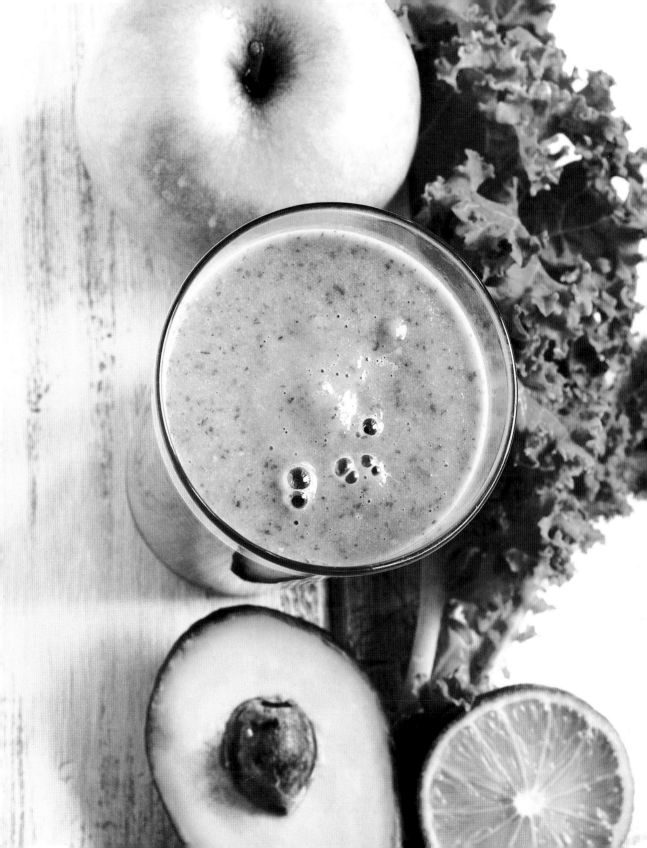

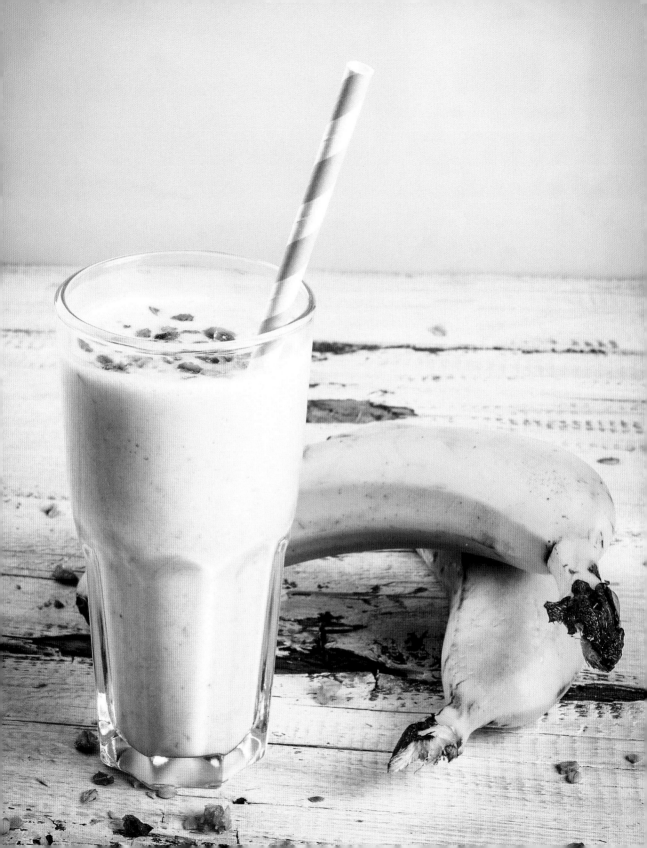

# Protein shake

A protein shake is something I look forward to just about every day. I only got into them in the past year because before I had always associated protein with bodybuilders and people who wanted to gain muscle. But now I know that protein is essential for repair after a workout and works well for me in moderation. I have one scoop of protein powder in a shake every day to help repair my muscles. And the fact that these shakes taste like a milkshake is a bonus.

   I should also mention how much I love my blender – I get so much use out of it. I actually have two, one in Dublin and one in London, because I can't be without them.

1 scoop vanilla protein (I go for a whey protein that is low in sugar and carbs)
handful of ice
1 small tsp organic peanut butter
1 banana
240ml unsweetened almond milk

Throw everything into a blender and whizz it around. It's so quick and simple to put together and makes a great mid-morning snack.

# LUNCH

I have a few lunch recipes that I make when I'm in a rush – nothing new there. They are super healthy and tasty and also quick!

## Salmon couscous

I love salmon and it is so easy to cook. Couscous is a healthy, light alternative to potatoes (even though I think sweet potatoes can be really good and keep you full).

1 salmon darne or fillet
1 lemon
half a packet of Mediterranean couscous
¼ pack halloumi cheese
bag of spinach
garlic, salt and pepper to taste

1. Preheat the oven to 180°C.
2. Place the salmon in some tinfoil and squeeze half the lemon juice on it. Wrap the tinfoil, but not too tightly.
3. Put the couscous in a bowl and pour in enough boiling water to come up a couple of centimetres above it. Cover with a tea towel.
4. Cook the salmon in the oven for 15 to 20 minutes. If you want a slightly crispy skin, grill the top for a minute.
5. Slice the halloumi. Pour a little olive oil into a frying pan and fry the cheese lightly on each side until cooked. Remove it from the pan and let it rest on a plate.
6. Crush the garlic. Then, using the same frying pan, cook the garlic and spinach until wilted. Add a sprinkle of salt and pepper.
7. Serve the salmon with the halloumi on top, on a bed of couscous, with the spinach and garlic on the side.

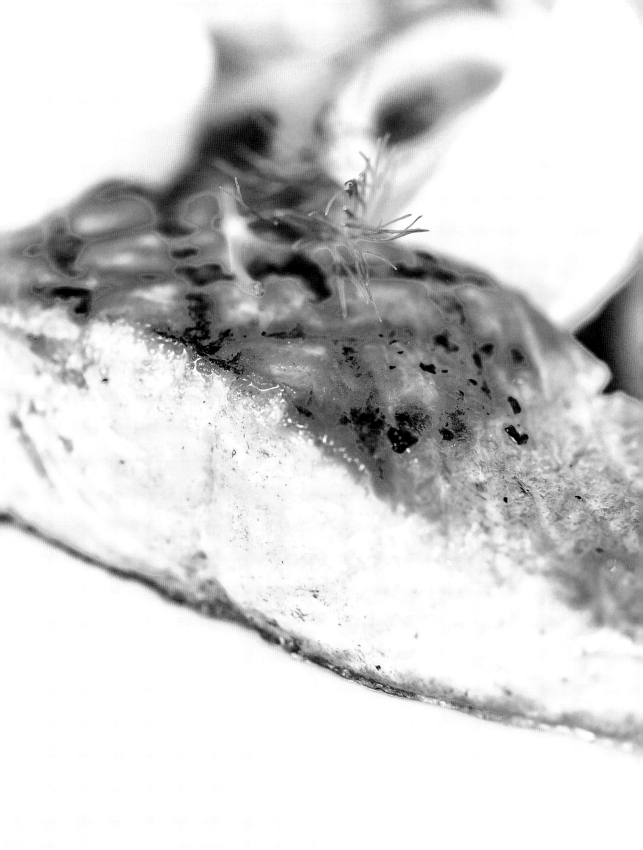

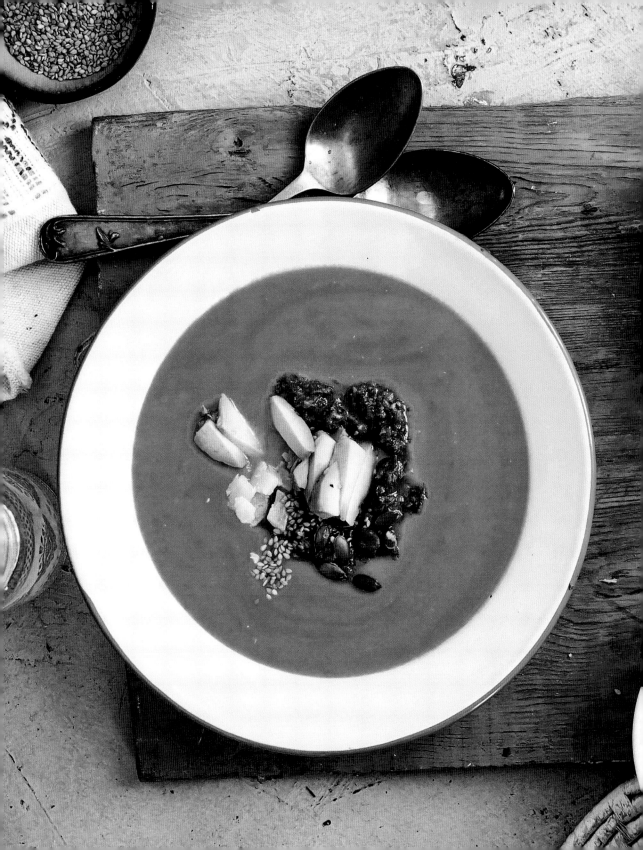

# Curried sweet potato and squash soup*

This is a wholesome, warming soup rich in Vitamin A.

3 sweet potatoes
1kg butternut squash
100g chopped onions
3 cloves garlic
900ml chicken stock
1 tbsp curry powder (to taste)
1 tbsp olive oil

1.  Cut the sweet potatoes and squash into approximately 1-inch squares.
2.  In a saucepan, fry the onion and garlic lightly before adding the chicken stock, sweet potatoes and squash. For a thick soup, add the stock until it barely covers the mixture. (Add curry powder now if desired.)
3.  Bring the mixture to a boil and cook until the sweet potato and squash are soft.
4.  Using a hand blender, puree until smooth.

(Vogue: If I'm feeling fancy, I'll add something on top – some nuts and seeds, or a bit of pesto.)

# Rice salad

This is definitely my favourite of my mom's salads. I have it with rocket and it's even better if I have leftover chicken from dinner. I have yet to master making it as well as my mom – when she gave me the recipe, she was quite vague about how much of each ingredient to use, so I go by taste!

1 ½ cups wild rice
1 white onion
1 tin sweetcorn
1 packet dried cranberries (I love these so sometimes use two)

For the dressing:
mayonnaise
curry paste or powder
mango chutney
a drizzle of vinegar (how much is really down to taste so start with a small drizzle and adjust to suit).

1.  Cook the rice, drain and leave in your serving bowl to cool.
2.  Make the dressing (you can do this while the rice is cooling). Put the mayonnaise into a bowl and then add the other ingredients. Taste as you go to make sure the flavour is how you like it. You need to make sure you have enough to coat the rice – none of it should be left dry.
3.  Chop the onion, then add it, the drained sweetcorn and the cranberries to the rice when it has cooled.
4.  Add the dressing to the rice mix and give it a really good stir. If I'm feeding a group of  people, I leave it in a big bowl at the table for them to help themselves.

# Spinach salad*

A very simple salad, full of iron, with a great balance of crunchy, tart and sweet tastes.

250g spinach
150g blueberries
200g feta cheese
100g cranberries
100g nuts and seeds mix
3 tbsp balsamic vinegar
1 tbsp olive oil

1. Rinse and dry the spinach and blueberries.
2. Cut the feta cheese into small pieces.
3. Combine everything together and toss lightly with balsamic vinegar and olive oil. This salad is lovely served with grilled salmon!

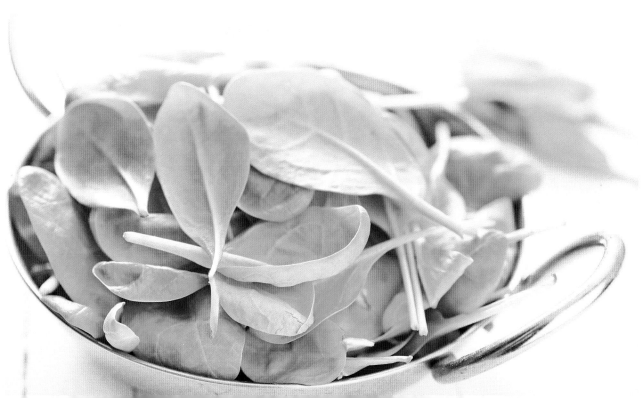

# Bulgar salad

1 bag bulgur wheat

1 bunch scallions

1 bag pine nuts

2 packets of semi-sundried tomatoes (save the oil for the dressing – see below)

1 packet dried cranberries

1 block soft goat's cheese

Dressing:

200ml olive oil

50ml balsamic vinegar

Oil from semi-sundried tomatoes

Salt and pepper

1 tsp pesto

1tsp French mustard

1.   Put the bulgur wheat in a bowl and add hot water so that the water level is approx half an inch above the grain. Then cover the bowl with a tea towel and leave to soak until the water is absorbed (approx 30 mins).

2.   Toast the pine nuts in the oven – spread on a roasting tray and cook at 180°C (160°C fan) for 5-10 minutes until they're golden brown. (Can also toast on a dry frying pan for approx 3 minutes – but make sure to shake the pan frequently, or the nuts will burn!)

3.   Wash and chop the scallions, then fry them until soft. Leave to the side.

4.   Mix the dressing ingredients together in a bowl, adding salt and pepper to taste

5.   Chop the goat's cheese into cubes, and halve the tomatoes.

6.   When ready, drain the excess water from the bulgur wheat.

7.   Add the cheese, pine nuts, cranberries, onions and tomatoes to the bulgur wheat and then add the dressing. Mix thoroughly. Garnish with mint if desired.

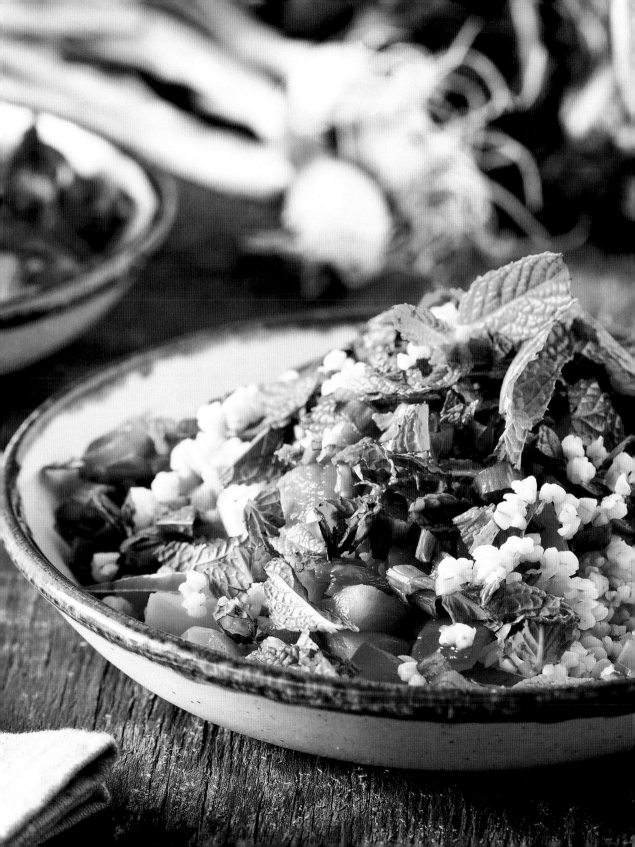

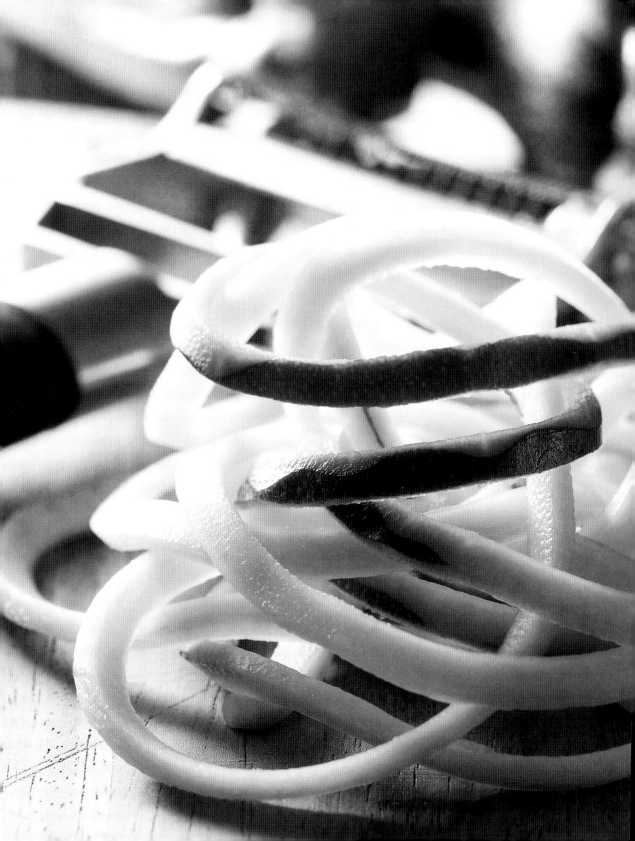

# DINNER

## Courgetti with arrabiata sauce

4 courgettes
4 cloves garlic
1 large white onion
2 red chillies
2 jars passata
handful of fresh basil
2 tbsp mixed herbs

1. If you have a spiralizer, use it to make your courgetti. I'm not in the habit of lying, so I will tell you that I always buy my courgetti in the supermarket!
2. Finely chop the garlic, onion and chillies – I always remove the chilli seeds too, as I don't like it too spicy.
3. Add a drop of olive oil to a pot and let it heat up.
4. Add the garlic, chillies and onion and allow to cook for two minutes.
5. Then add the passata and allow to simmer for five minutes.
6. Add the basil and mixed herbs and allow to simmer again for twenty minutes and, voilà, you have your arrabiata sauce.
7. Sometimes I heat my courgetti by frying lightly in oil but more often than not, I'll heat in the sauce and serve.

# Green curry

*Serves 6*

I love green curry – it's my takeaway order of choice – but I found a way of making an even healthier version that's just as nice and is ideal for freezing. It's loaded with vegetables too, so it's an easy way to get your greens in. You can mix up the veg using whatever you fancy – mushrooms, peas, peppers etc. And you can substitute the chicken with prawns, beef or tofu, depending on your preference.

I always make sure to buy a good Thai curry paste. Even though I've suggested an amount to use, you should taste as you cook to make sure it's right for you. Don't go too wild with it, though, because it can be seriously spicy. But if spice is what you like, you can pop in a chilli too!

1 large packet of green beans
3 courgettes
2 fresh kaffir lime leaves
handful of basil leaves
1 tbsp coconut oil
garlic (I usually buy garlic in a tube and use half of it)
1 rounded tbsp Thai green curry paste
3 cans coconut milk (I use two full fat and one low fat)
2 tsp Thai fish sauce
4–5 chicken breasts, chopped into bite-size pieces
boiled brown rice, to serve

1.  Trim and halve the green beans, halve the courgettes and slice them into chunks and shred the kaffir lime leaves and basil.
2.  In a wok or large frying pan, heat the coconut oil until it is very hot.
3.  Drop in the garlic and cook until it's golden, which should take about 20 seconds.

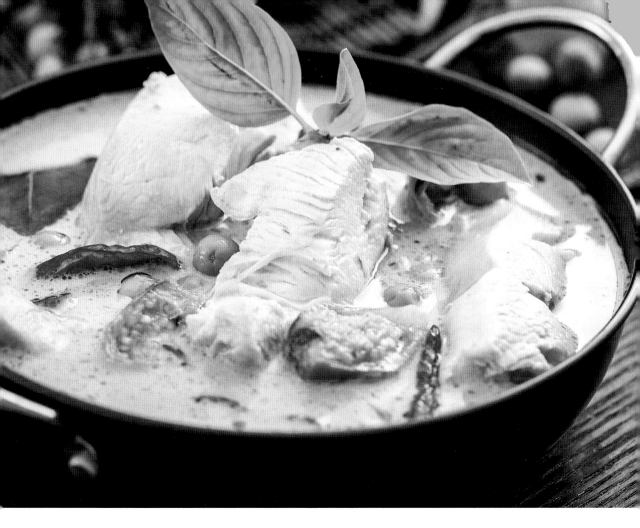

4. Spoon in the curry paste and stir it around for a few seconds to begin to cook the spices and release all the flavours.

5. Pour in the coconut milk and let it come to a boil – always shake the can before you open it.

6. Pour in the fish sauce (this comes in a glass bottle and stinks if you spill it – I learned this the hard way after smashing a bottle of the stuff).

7. Add the pieces of chicken and leave to simmer for about ten minutes.

8. Add the green beans, courgettes, kaffir lime leaves and basil and stir through.

9. Simmer for 20 to 25 mins, until the veg has softened.

10. Serve with brown rice.

# Chicken stir-fry

*Serves 2*

One of the best meals you can eat to ensure you get plenty of vegetables is a stir-fry. It tastes so nice and you can chuck in any vegetables you like and any meat or fish, depending on your preference. I usually like to use chicken or prawns, although I sometimes add fillet steak – red meat is such a great source of iron.

   The preparation is the longest part of making this meal, as there is a lot of chopping, but it only takes ten minutes to cook when you have everything ready. I would only make a stir-fry on the night I plan to eat it – it doesn't really keep well.

2 chicken breasts
2 peppers (green and yellow are my favourites, but you can use any colour)
1 red onion
half a head of broccoli
1 bok choy
2 cloves garlic
1 tbsp sesame oil
1 tsp Chinese five-spice powder
light soy sauce
cooked brown rice or noodles, to serve
sprinkling of toasted sesame seeds, to garnish (optional)

1.   Slice the chicken breasts and leave to one side.
2.   Slice the peppers, roughly chop the onion and separate the broccoli. Put them all in a bowl and set to one side.
3.   Slice the bok choy and leave in a separate bowl.
4.   Add the sesame oil to a wok and allow it to heat.
5.   Chop the garlic, add and stir it to ensure it doesn't burn.

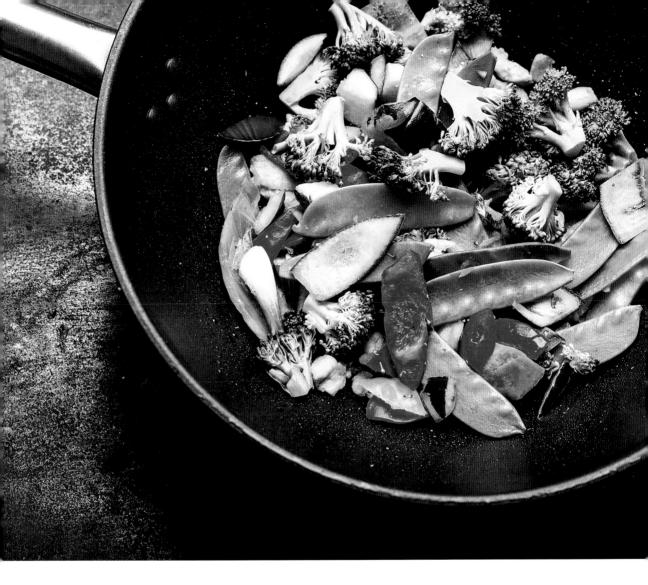

6. Add the chicken breasts and cook until there is no pink meat visible.
7. Add the peppers, onion and broccoli, and stir.
8. Add the five-spice powder and a dash of soy sauce.
9. Add the bok choy at the very end, as it cooks really quickly. I never let the vegetables go too soft as I prefer them to have a little crunch.
10. Serve with a small portion of brown rice or noodles, sprinkled with the sesame seeds (if using).

# Chilli con carne

*Serves 8*

I always have some chilli ready to go in my freezer because it's an easy, healthy meal, so I cook a lot of it in batches. It's great for dinner parties too.

I add carrots to this recipe, though they are not essential, but I think they bulk up the chilli and it's an easy way to add more veg to your diet. Try to use minced beef or even minced turkey that has a low fat percentage – sometimes I use steak pieces chopped up if I'm bored of mince.

2 medium onions

4 sticks celery

3 peppers (any colour)

4 carrots (optional)

1 tbsp coconut oil

4 cloves garlic (or half a tube of garlic paste)

1kg minced beef

2 tsp chilli powder

2 tsp ground cumin

2 tsp ground paprika

salt and pepper

1 tin red kidney beans

1 tin chickpeas

3–4 tins chopped tomatoes

boiled brown rice and green beans or spinach, to serve

1.  Roughly chop the onions, celery, peppers and carrots (if using).
2.  Add the coconut oil to a pan over a medium heat and let it melt.
3.  Add the garlic and cook for 20 seconds.

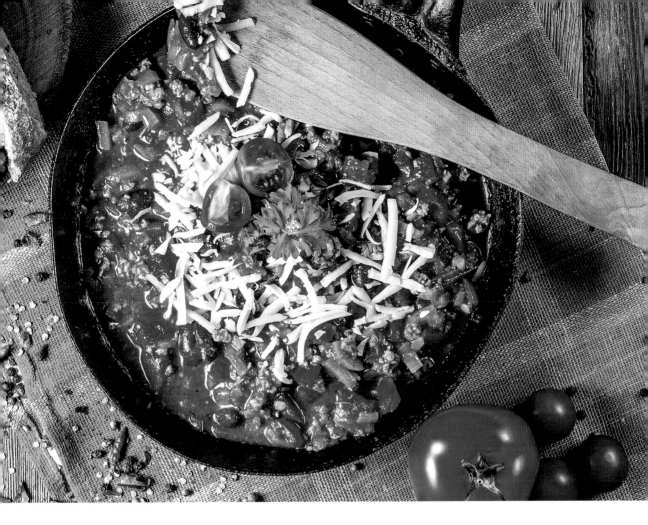

4. Add the beef and cook until browned, then throw in all the spices and salt and pepper.

5. Add the onions, celery, peppers and carrots (if using) and cook for another five minutes.

6. Add three tins of chopped tomatoes and allow to simmer for 20 minutes.

7. Add in the kidney beans and chickpeas and, if you like your chilli with a little extra sauce, the fourth can of chopped tomatoes. Allow to simmer for another 15 minutes. I usually wait until the next day to eat my chilli as I think it needs a few hours to sit, but you can eat it straight away if you want to.

8. Serve with brown rice and some green beans or spinach on the side too.

# Ratatouille

*Serves 6*

This goes really well with steak, fish or grilled chicken. It's a great low-carb option for dinner and tastes so good. If I want to add good carbs, I will have some sweet potato wedges with it. A traditional ratatouille has aubergines as well as courgettes, but I don't like them much, so I add extra courgettes instead. You can use aubergines too, though, if you prefer.

2 aubergines (optional)
4 courgettes (if you are using aubergines, 3 courgettes is enough)
2 peppers, any colour
1 chilli
5 tbsp olive oil
small tub cherry tomatoes
large bunch of fresh basil
1 large onion
3 cloves garlic
1 tbsp balsamic vinegar
1 tsp agave syrup
2 tins chopped tomatoes

1. If you are using them, cut the aubergines in half lengthways and then into chunks.
2. Cut the courgettes into quite thick slices. Cut the peppers into bite-size chunks. Finely slice and deseed the chilli.
3. Pour 2 tbsp of olive oil into a frying pan and add the aubergines. Cook until soft, then set aside in a bowl.
4. Add another tablespoon of oil and fry the courgettes for 5 minutes, until they are golden, then put them in the bowl with the aubergines.

5.  Add another tablespoon of oil and fry the peppers until soft, then add them to the bowl with the aubergines and courgettes.
6.  Add the final tablespoon of oil and fry the cherry tomatoes until soft, then add them to the bowl with the other vegetables. (Don't overcook the vegetables at this stage, as they have more cooking time left.)
7.  Tear up the basil leaves and set aside.
8.  Chop the onion and cook in the pan for 5 minutes.
9.  Crush the garlic and add to the onion, frying for another minute.
10. Stir in the vinegar and agave syrup, then tip in the tinned tomatoes and half the basil.
11. Add the aubergines, courgettes, cherry tomatoes and peppers to the pan. Add salt and pepper to taste and cook for 5 minutes.
12. Sprinkle the remainder of the basil on top and serve.

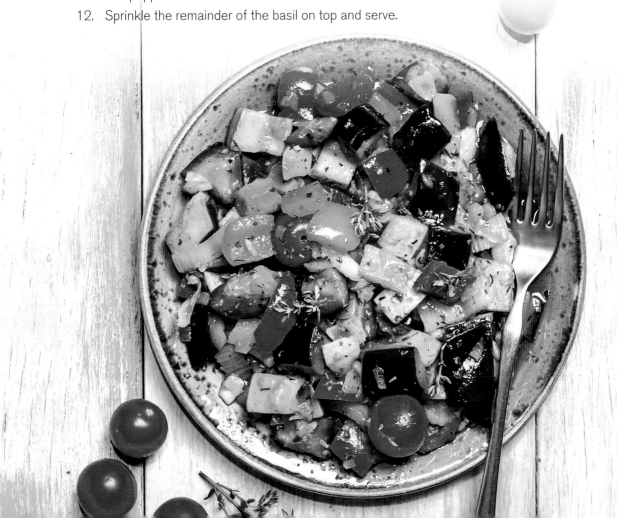

# Yuk sung

*Serves 4*

Despite the name, this is not yuk! It's one of my favourite dishes when I go out for a Chinese, so I started making it at home too – and it's super easy.

I don't add in the crispy rice because it makes it a little bit less healthy. And, traditionally, the recipe includes minced pork but I also change this up because I don't really like the smell of minced pork and minced chicken works just as well – it's just harder to find. My mom makes this recipe all the time, so I stole it from her (again)!

2 cloves garlic
2 chillies
root ginger (use as much or as little as you like, but 3cm is normally enough)
2 stalks celery
2 spring onions
1 tin water chestnuts
1 iceberg lettuce (to serve)
a good drizzle of sesame oil for frying
500g minced pork or chicken

**Sauce**

| | |
|---|---|
| 2 tbsp dark soy sauce | 2 tbsp dry sherry |
| 4 tbsp oyster sauce | 2 tsp sugar |

1.  I like to get all my ingredients chopped and ready to go so when it comes to the cooking part I just have to throw it all in. Chop the garlic. Deseed the chillies and chop as finely as the garlic. Slice the ginger very thinly. Chop the celery into quite small chunks. Roughly chop the spring onions. Drain and quarter the water chestnuts.
2.  Wash the lettuce and separate the leaves so they are ready to serve.

3.   Mix the sauce ingredients in a bowl and leave to one side. You will only add half of this to the mince when cooking. (I am a big fan of sauces so I always make extra and use the remaining half to add to my lettuce wrap when it's cooked. Not the healthiest but worth it!)

4.   Add the sesame oil to a frying pan and after about 20 seconds add the garlic, chilli, ginger, celery, spring onions, and water chestnuts and fry for a few minutes.

5.   Add the meat and cook until brown, pouring in your sauce halfway through.

6.   Place some of the cooked meat mixture in a lettuce leaf (now's the time for me to add some leftover sauce!) and serve.

7.   As with lots of my meals, I usually double the ingredients so I have some left over, as yuk sung still tastes nice after two days and it saves me cooking more!

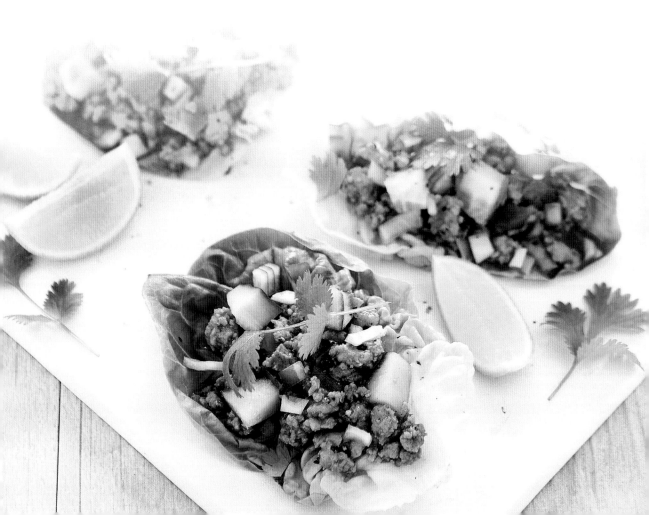

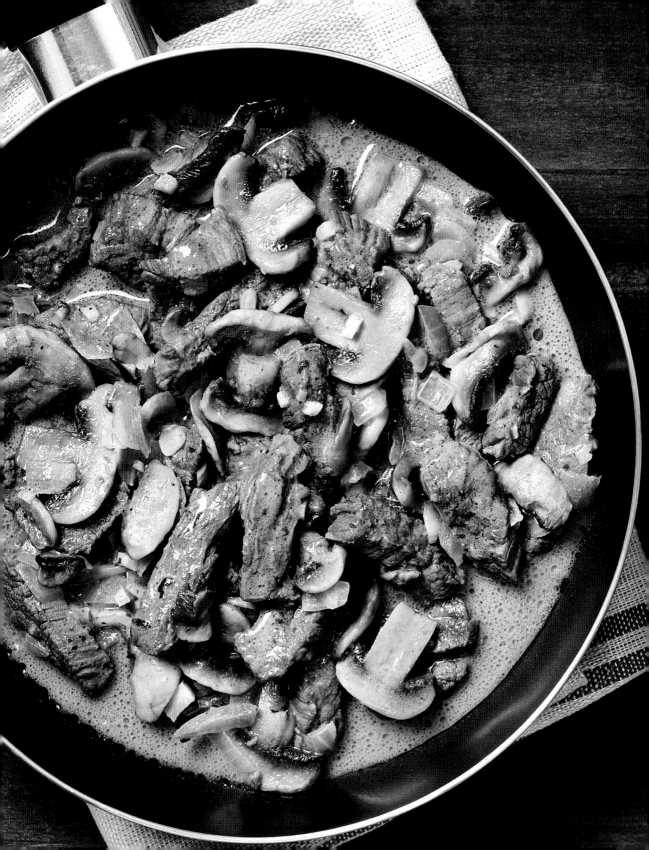

# Beef stroganoff

*Serves 6–8*

This is another recipe I've stolen from my mom, after ordering beef stroganoff out at lunch one day and being really disappointed because I'm used to Mom's recipe and how good it tastes. Now, this is not my healthiest recipe but it is beyond delicious. I serve it with rice but you could use potatoes or pasta instead.

1½ lb fillet of beef (I always use the fillet because it's the nicest part)
2 white onions
3 cloves garlic
¼ of a 454g block of butter (if you want to be healthier you can use olive oil)
a good dose of paprika
fresh chillies to taste (optional)
1 packet button mushrooms, cleaned
300ml sour cream
juice of 1 lemon
salt and pepper to taste
brown rice to serve

1. Cut the beef into small strips. Chop the onions, and crush the garlic and slice the mushrooms.
2. Melt the butter (or olive oil) in a pan and add the paprika, onions and garlic.
3. Cook until the onions soften.
4. If you are using the chillies for a little more spice, chop them and add to the pan along with the sliced mushrooms and cook for a few minutes.
5. Add the beef and brown on each side.
6. Pour in the sour cream and lemon juice and cook for a few minutes. Don't let the beef cook too much as it will get tough.
7. Serve with cooked rice.

# One-step salmon and vegetables*

*Serves 1*

This simple, healthy one-step dish can be adapted to serve as many (or few) people as you want.

140g piece of salmon
100g asparagus
½ red pepper
½ yellow pepper
100g cherry vine tomatoes, halved
olive oil
2 tbsp pesto

1.  Preheat the oven to 190°C.
2.  Lightly toss all the vegetables and the salmon in some olive oil. You can add any vegetables you want to this, but be conscious of cooking time. For example, potatoes or squash may need to be pre-cooked.
3.  Take a large piece of parchment-lined aluminium foil, add the vegetables (foil side out) and place the salmon on top.
4.  Brush the salmon with the pesto.
5.  Fold up the foil into a package, place in the oven and cook for 20 minutes.

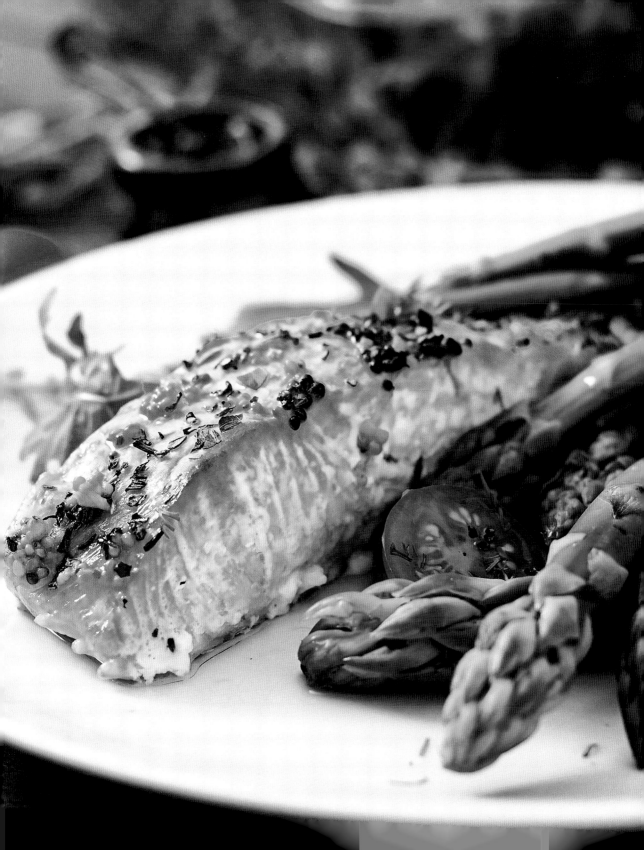

# Turkey lasagne*

A family favourite adapted for turkey mince, full of calcium and fibre. If you want to make the recipe wheat-free, simply swap the noodles for a wheat-free version.

200g courgettes
450g minced turkey
2 tsp olive oil
200ml chicken stock
400g passata
150g double-concentrated tomato puree
mixed herbs
600g low-fat cottage cheese
150ml skimmed milk
wholewheat lasagne noodles
200g light mozzarella cheese

1. Preheat the oven to 200°C.
2. Cut the courgettes into small pieces, combine with the turkey and fry on medium heat in olive oil.
3. Add in the chicken stock to moisten the meat.
4. Once the turkey has partially cooked (whitened on the outside) and the chicken stock has absorbed into the meat, add the passata, tomato paste, and mixed herbs (to taste).
5. Cook on medium heat until turkey is fully cooked.
6. Mix the cottage cheese and milk in a bowl.
7. In a large lasagne dish, put half of the meat mixture, cover with a layer of noodles and then a layer of half the cottage cheese mix. Repeat. Top with grated mozzarella.
8. Cook in the oven for 20 minutes or until the cheese crisps. Allow to rest for 15 minutes before cutting and serving.

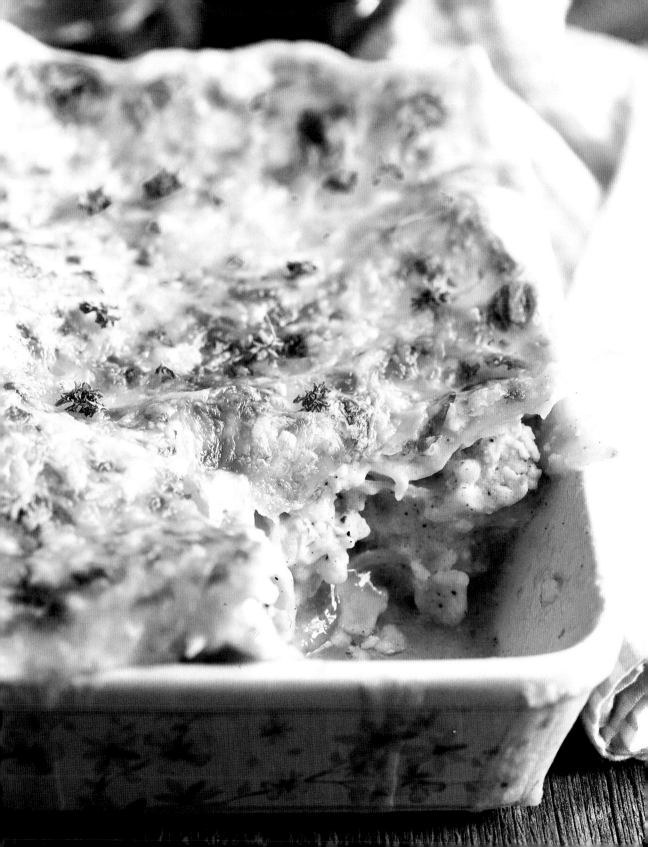

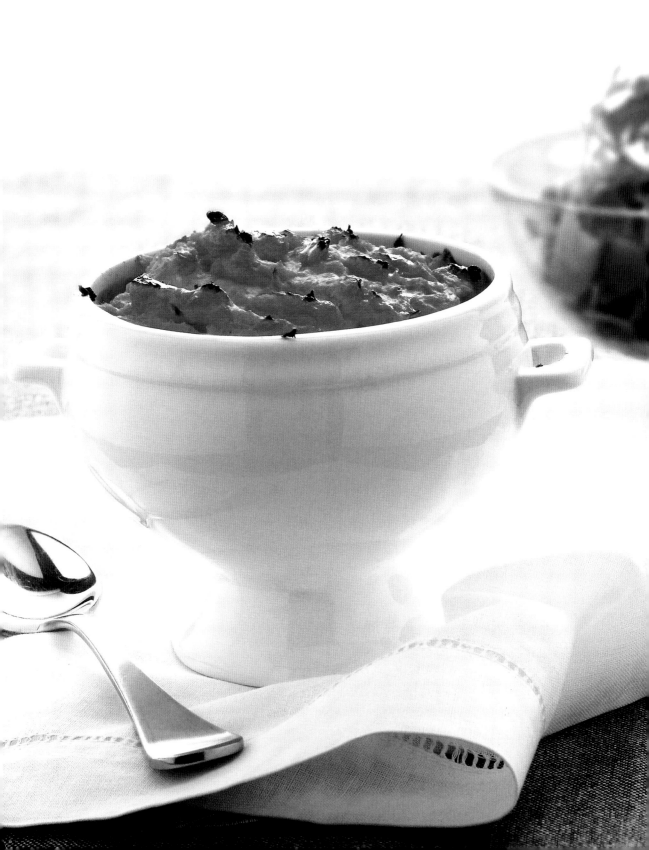

# Sweet potato turkey cottage pie*

A healthy, protein-packed take on a classic dish, topped with sweet potato for added goodness.

1kg sweet potatoes
75g carrots
450g minced turkey
olive oil
200ml chicken stock
1 tsp flour
75g peas
1 tsp cinnamon
salt and pepper
50g olive-oil-based spread

1. Preheat the oven to 190°C.
2. Peel and dice the sweet potatoes and carrots. Place the sweet potatoes in a saucepan of boiling water over a medium heat and cook until soft.
3. Meanwhile, fry the turkey mince in a little olive oil over a medium heat until starting to cook on the outside.
4. Add the chicken stock and flour and continue to stir as the juices thicken.
5. Add the diced carrots and peas and fry until just cooked (the carrots should still have some bite).
6. When the sweet potatoes are cooked, drain and mash them with the cinnamon, salt and pepper (to taste) and spread.
7. Place the turkey mixture in a 10x6-inch baking dish and top with the sweet potatoes. Bake for 15 minutes.

# Having People Over

I love having friends around and will usually do one of my curries or chillies which I can prepare before they arrive. This leaves me plenty of time for socialising with them. And if I'm being really nice to my friends, I'll make the prawn dish on page 116. I live by the sea in Ireland where the most amazing fish is available. If the weather is good – even just a little bit warm – I'll try to do a barbecue. I make baby potatoes tossed in butter and salt, as well as some salads, as side dishes. I lay out bowls of everything on the table and let everyone serve themselves.

## Burgers

I love a good burger. My recipe is tasty *and* healthy, so I don't need to feel guilty while enjoying it. These freeze well too so I always make a big batch of them.

2 red peppers
1 large white onion (I usually buy the pre-chopped ones because I despise chopping onions!)
1kg mince (use a mince with a low fat percentage)
1 large egg
squeeze of ketchup
salt and pepper
1 tbsp chilli flakes
1 tbsp mixed herbs
2 cloves garlic

1. Preheat the oven to 200°C.
2. Finely chop the peppers, garlic and onion.
3. Put the mince into a big bowl and scrunch it (with clean hands) to break it down.
4. Add the rest of the ingredients and mix thoroughly with your hands.
5. Scoop out a small amount of the mixture and roll in your hands. Then flatten it and leave to the side.

6. If you're not barbequing them, fry the burgers quickly on each side till browned, then put them on a baking tray. Bake until they are cooked the way you like them. Bake for about 20 minutes until cooked through.

7. I always serve my burgers with some avocado, tomato, rocket, goat's cheese and a little drizzle of sweet chilli sauce.

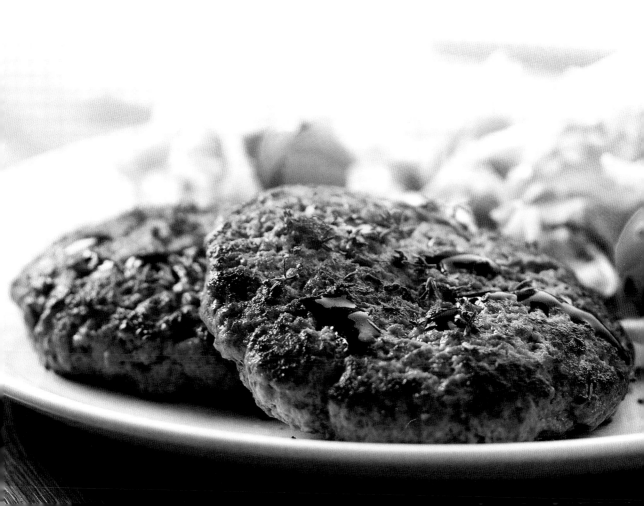

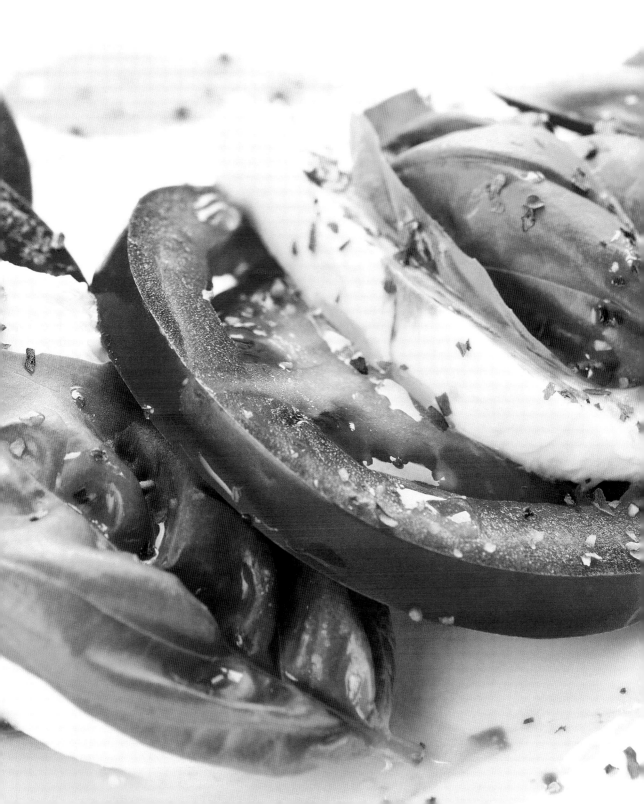

# Caprese salad

This is probably one of the easiest salads to make but it's so delicious – I always order it in restaurants too. I buy a good buffalo mozzarella and always use fresh basil (and plenty of it). Everybody loves this when I make it as a starter at dinner parties or as part of the barbecue spread. And anything with cheese is always a winner in my eyes!

2 balls mozzarella
full packet fresh basil
6 tomatoes
olive oil
black pepper

1. Slice the mozzarella and the tomatoes into fairly thick slices. Layer them on a plate.
2. Wash the basil, tear and sprinkle it on top.
3. Add a big drizzle of olive oil and then grind on some black pepper.

# Roasted sweet potato salad*

This is a great healthy alternative to traditional potato salads and is rich in vitamin A and calcium.

1½kg sweet potatoes
olive oil
salt and pepper
150g feta cheese
100g pine nuts
120g rocket
balsamic vinegar

1.  Preheat the oven to 200°C.
2.  Cut the sweet potato into small cubes, toss in olive oil and season with salt and pepper. Place on a baking sheet and bake for 45 minutes (or until fully cooked). Allow to cool.
3.  Mix the roasted sweet potato with the feta cheese and pine nuts.
4.  Place the rocket in a big bowl, with the sweet potato mix on top, and dress with balsamic vinegar and 2 tbsp olive oil.

(Vogue: Sometimes I add pomegranate seeds for a sweeter twist on the recipe.)

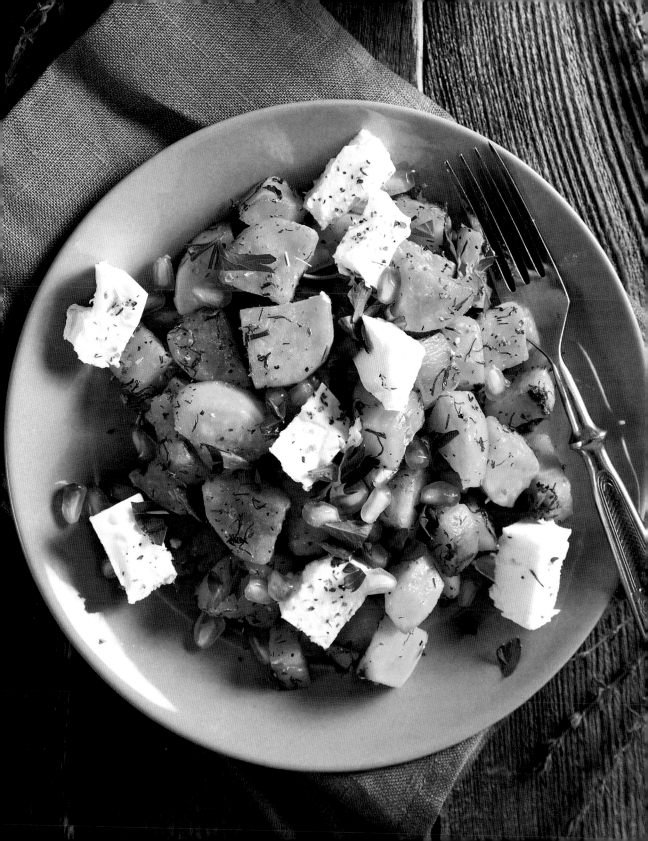

# Garlic prawns

These are my absolute favourite and make a great starter with crusty bread for a dinner party. They're really easy to make, once you've done the torturous task of getting the shell off the prawn. Don't use the small ones from the supermarket – you need really big prawns for this dish.

2 chillies
2 cloves garlic
approx. 220g of butter
20 large fresh prawns
1 glass white wine

1.  Deseed and finely chop the chillies and slice the garlic.
2.  Melt the butter in a frying pan – be careful not to let it burn.
3.  Add the chillies and garlic and fry for 30 seconds.
4.  Add the prawns and the wine and stir. The prawns should cook in about five minutes, so make sure you keep an eye on them – when they turn pink, they're done!
5.  Serve with some crusty bread to soak up the sauce.

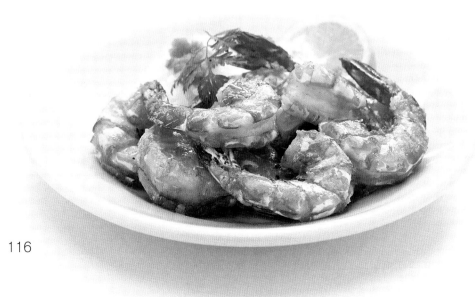

# Tandoori chicken

I have steak, sausages and chicken with every barbecue. I keep the sausages plain and just add a little bit of barbecue sauce to the steak, so I like to make my chicken nice and flavoursome. Serves 6.

1 large tub of plain yoghurt
tandoori paste
½ lemon
6 chicken breasts (thighs or drumsticks also work well)

1.  Put the yoghurt into a dish large enough to fit all the chicken.
2.  Mix the tandoori paste into the yoghurt – it will turn a nice orange colour. Do a taste test on this.
3.  Squeeze the juice of the lemon half into the yoghurt and mix thoroughly.
4.  Add the chicken to the mix and leave to marinate for a few hours.

If I don't cook this on the BBQ, I would bake it in a pre-heated oven at 180 degrees Celsius for 30–40 minutes until the chicken is cooked through. Whether you're cooking on a BBQ or in an oven, always make sure your chicken is cooked through.

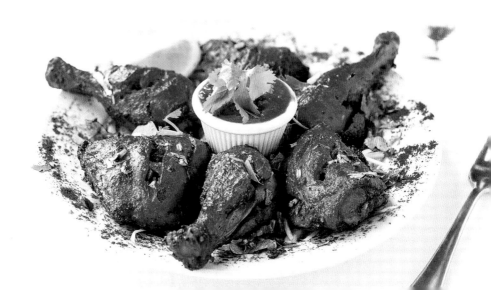

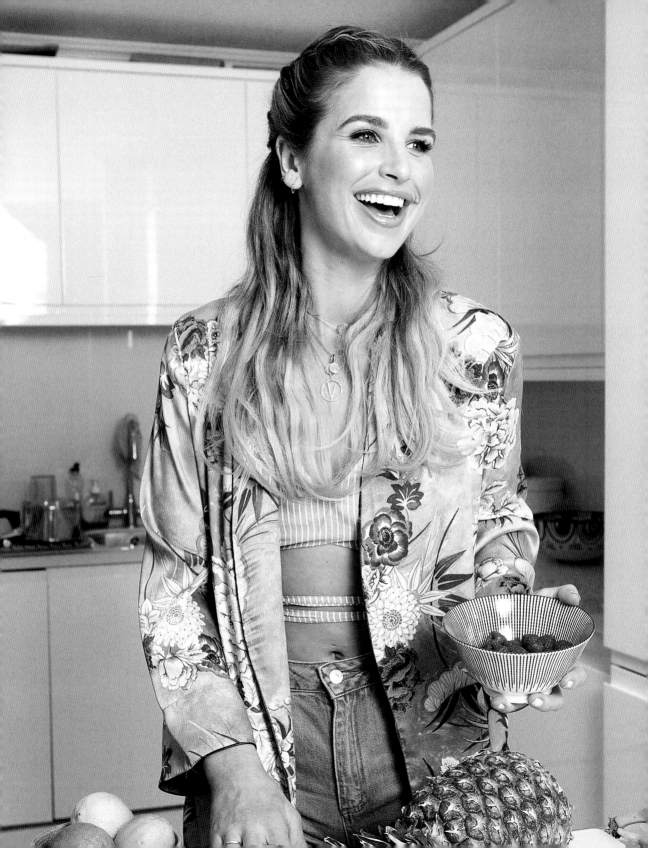

# SNACKS

## Chocolate peanut-butter protein bars

I am obsessed with these snack bars – personal trainer Erica Brennan gave me the recipe. They are really filling and I think they're as nice as Snickers – maybe even nicer! I eat these during the day with a cup of tea as a treat, but a healthy treat that keeps me full. I often make double portions and freeze half, so I always have some ready.

280g organic peanut butter
4tbsp honey
25g chocolate protein powder
25g gluten-free oats
2 tsp flaxseed mix
1 tsp cacao nibs

1. Put the peanut butter and honey into a bowl and heat in the microwave for 90 seconds.
2. Add the rest of the ingredients and stir.
3. Put in a container (I use a lunch box) and flatten it so it is spread evenly.
4. Leave in the fridge for a minimum of 30 minutes.
5. Boil the kettle, make herbal tea – matcha green tea is one of my favourites – cut your bars, eat and enjoy!

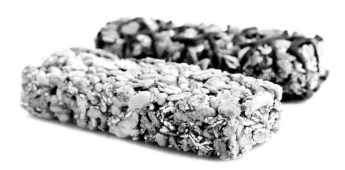

# Protein balls

I love having protein balls ready because they're another great snack you can have on the go and are full of good stuff!

½ cup sesame seeds
5–6 tbsp pumpkin seeds
1 cup dates (stoned)
¾ cup raw cacao powder
4–5 tsp organic crunchy peanut butter
4 tbsp melted coconut oil (you can add more if mixture is too dry)
handful mixed nuts (walnuts, pecans, hazelnuts, Brazils)
handful desiccated coconut

1.   Preheat oven to 200°C.
2.   Put the sesame seeds and pumpkin seeds on a baking tray and toast in the oven for 8–10 minutes, until browned.
3.   Meanwhile, put the dates, cacao powder, crunchy peanut butter, coconut oil, mixed nuts and desiccated coconut into a blender and blitz until it forms a dough.
4.   Take a small amount of the dough and roll it into a ball in your hands.
5.   Roll each ball in the toasted sesame and pumpkin seeds to coat them.
6.   Place the finished balls on a baking tray and put them in the freezer.
7.   After two hours, remove from the freezer and keep in the fridge.

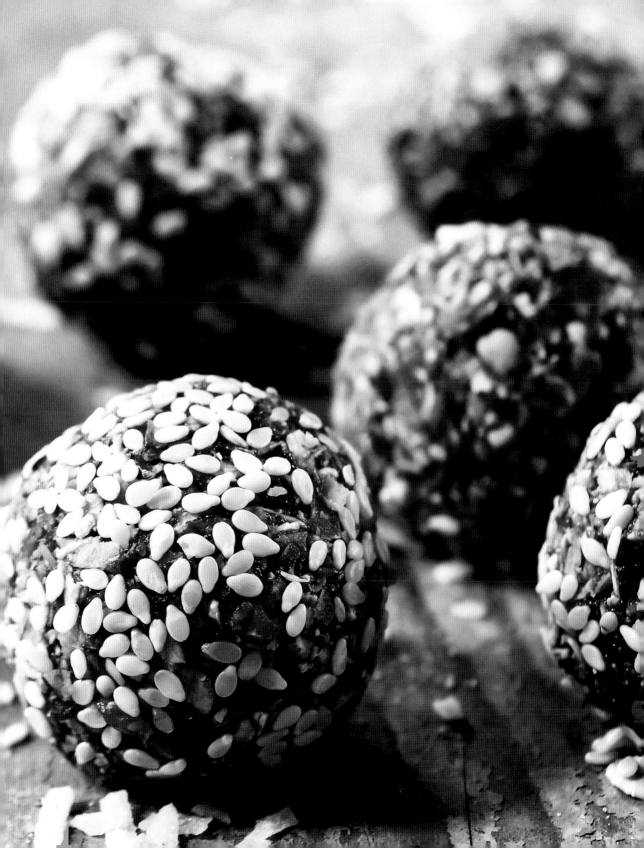

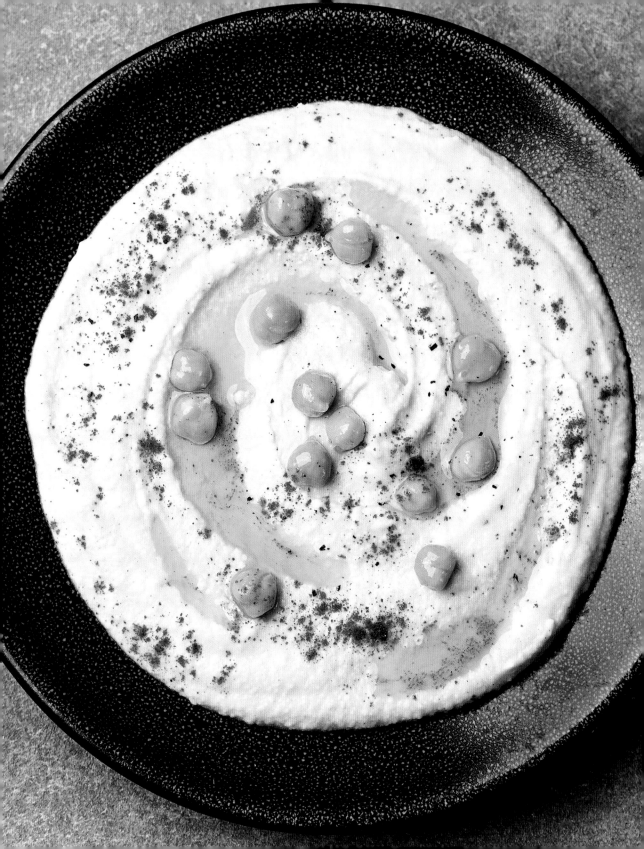

# Hummus

If you follow me on social media, you will have noticed my obsession with hummus. It's my favourite afternoon snack. If I don't have time to make it myself, I just buy one in the shop – but homemade is always nicer. And I'm always trying out new flavours, which is easy to do when you have the basic recipe. You can add roasted red peppers, piri-piri seasoning, sweet chilli sauce (I'm a big fan of this flavour) or jalapenos to make a spicy hummus – the possibilities are endless.

2 cans chickpeas
4 tbsp lemon juice
4 cloves garlic (I love garlic but you might want to use less)
2 tsp ground cumin
salt and pepper to taste
8 tbsp water
4 tbsp extra virgin olive oil
2 tsp paprika

1. Drain and wash the chickpeas.
2. Place all of the ingredients in a blender, add whatever seasoning or flavour you feel like and blitz until you have a nice creamy texture. I always taste a little and add more flavouring, salt or lemon juice if needed.

# Avocados for the win

I was trying to avoid including a million recipes for avocados, but I eat them every day so I couldn't really help myself. I only developed a taste for them when I moved to Australia, but now I'm addicted. They are so good for you, too. They are high in fat – but it's good fat that your body needs. Just don't eat a hundred in a day and you'll be fine!

Here are my top avocado recipes – along with the baked avocado for breakfast, these are the ones that I can't go without.

# Holy moly guacamole

I never buy guacamole in a shop – it just doesn't taste as nice or as fresh as when I make it myself. Don't leave the mix hanging around too long, as it tends to go a bit brown in colour (it will still taste fine, but it doesn't look as good).

4 ripe avocados
1 red onion
8 cherry tomatoes
1 lime
salt and pepper to taste

1.	Halve and stone the avocados. Scoop the flesh out with a spoon, put it in a bowl and mash.
2.	Chop the red onion and tomatoes finely and add to the avocado.
3.	Squeeze the juice of the lime into the mix and add salt and pepper to taste.
4.	Mix it all up and serve.

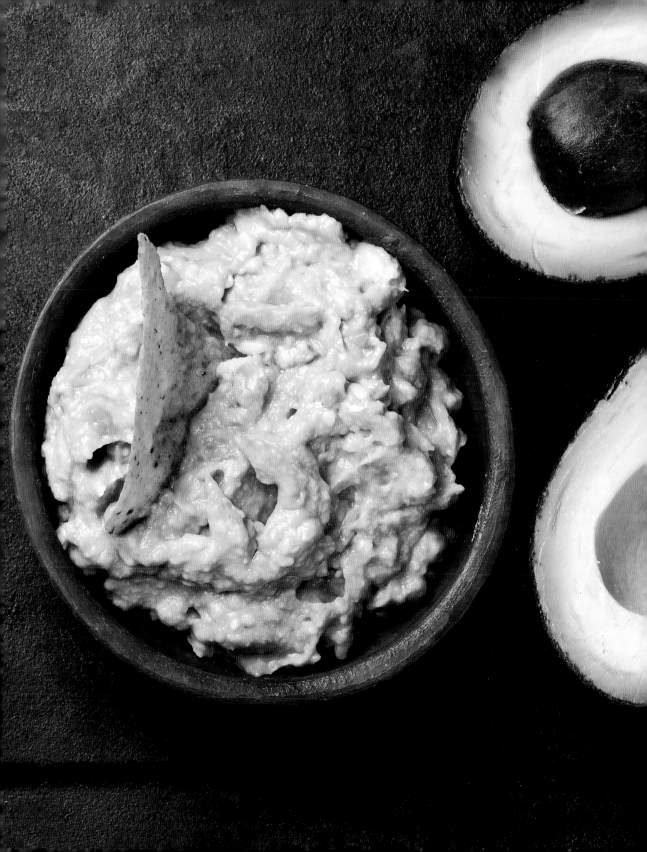

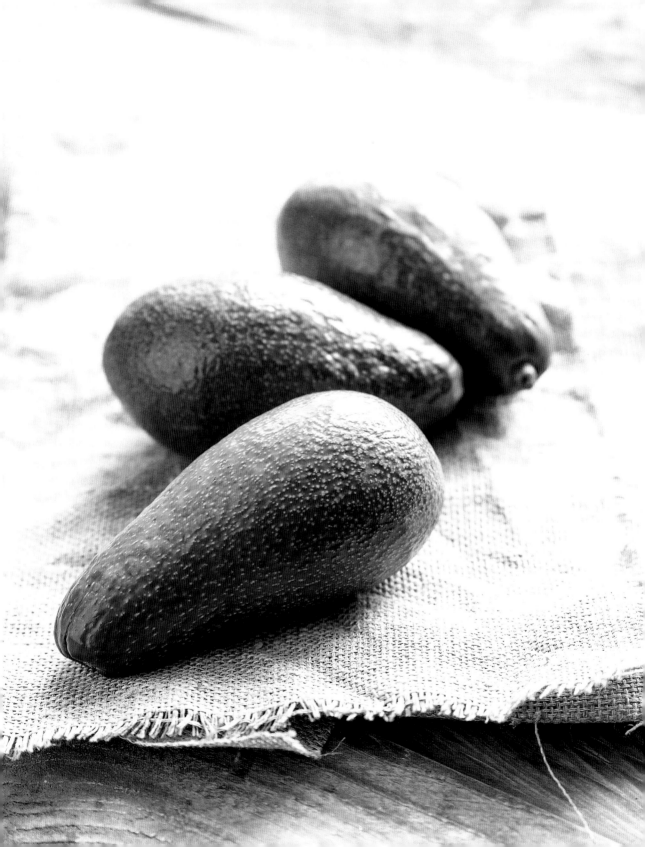

# Avo chips

I love chips as much as everyone else – I'm assuming everyone does, and if you don't, I don't understand you! I am not saying my avocado chips taste like those from a chipper, but they are great as a side dish or to serve as canapés while your guests are having the chats over a drink. I serve them with a garlic aioli to dip into.

4 avocados
½ cup flour
3 eggs
1¼ cups polenta
1 tsp garlic powder
1 tsp chilli powder
salt and pepper
low-fat cooking spray

1. Preheat oven to 200°C.
2. Cover a baking tray with greaseproof paper and spray with low-fat cooking spray.
3. Halve and stone the avocados and cut into fairly thick slices.
4. Coat each slice with flour, shaking off any excess.
5. In a small bowl, whisk the eggs.
6. In a separate bowl, mix the polenta, garlic powder, chilli powder, salt and pepper.
7. Dip each flour-coated avocado slice in the egg.
8. Then dip each one in the polenta mix.
9. Place coated avocados in a single layer on the prepared baking sheet.
10. Spray with some low-fat cooking spray.
11. Cook for 15–20 minutes until browned.

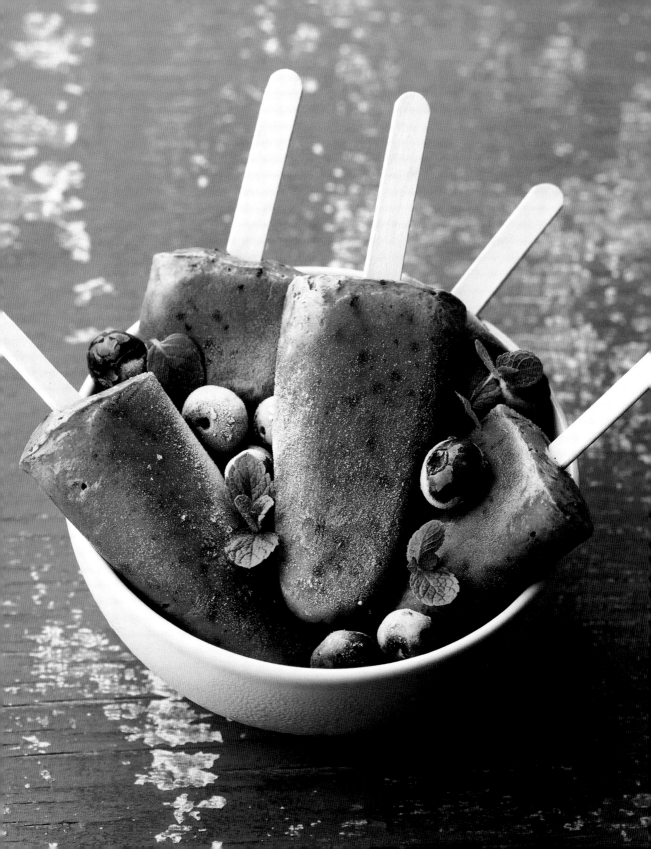

# TREATS!

## Ice-pops

I don't know why but at night-time I always want something sweet to eat. I can eat healthily all day, but when it gets to eight o'clock, I go diving for the chocolate. I try my best to stick to my routine of eating healthily during the week, though, so I came up with this alternative that is sweet *and* healthy – best of both worlds.

1 punnet strawberries
1 punnet blueberries
1 lime
1 cup coconut water

1. Wash the strawberries and blueberries and remove the stalks from the strawberries.
2. Put the berries into a blender with the coconut water and squeeze the juice of the lime on top.
3. Blend until smooth, then pour into ice-pop moulds.
4. Leave them in the freezer overnight, and then eat them all!

# Sugar-free banana muffins*

*Makes 12*

These are a delicious, energy-filled snack that work great for a pre-exercise burst of energy. They have no added sugar and are high in fibre.

3 ripe bananas
100g sugar-free stewed apple
50g raisins
150g rolled oats
1 egg
100g wholemeal (or seeded) flour
2 tsp cinnamon (to taste)
1 tsp baking powder
pinch of salt
250ml milk (you might need less)

1.  Preheat oven to 190°C.
2.  Using a potato masher, mash the bananas until there are no lumps.
3.  Add apple sauce, raisins, oats, egg, flour, cinnamon, baking powder and salt.
4.  Add the milk until the mixture is a smooth dropping consistency.
5.  Line a 12-cup muffin tin with paper cases and divide the mixture evenly between the cups. Bake for 20 minutes.

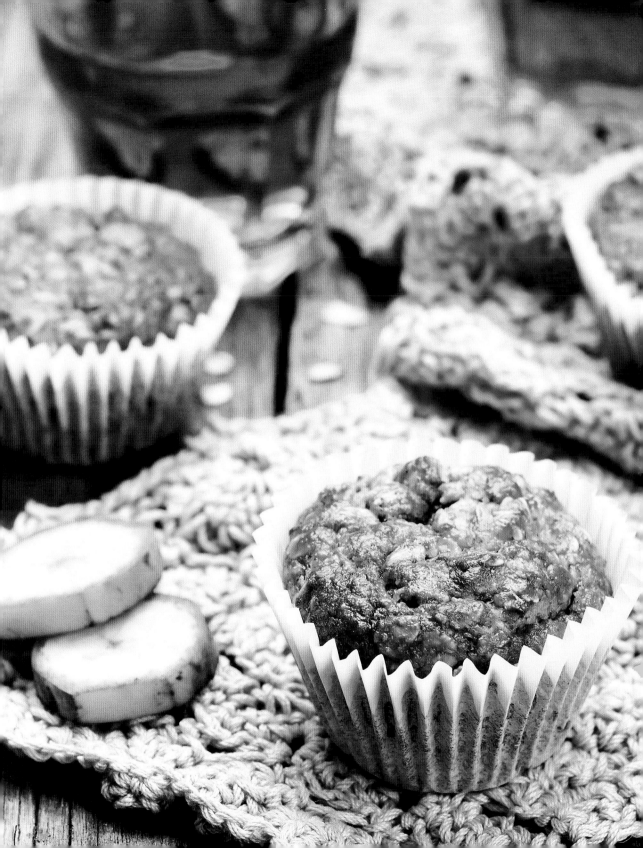

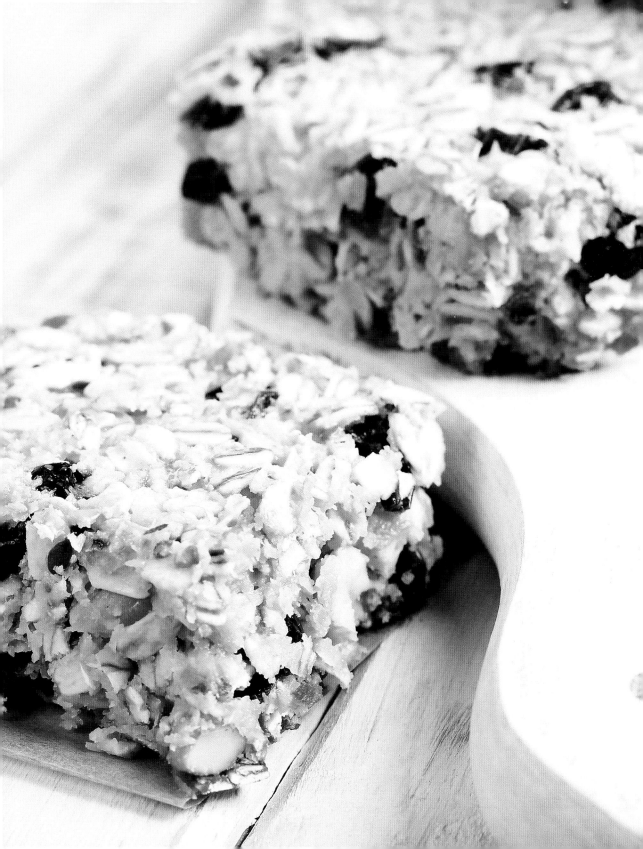

# Apricot and cranberry sugar-free flapjacks

These are an easy-to-make, healthy alternative to the sugar-laden commercial versions.

200g Medjool dates
100g sugar-free stewed apple
3 over-ripe bananas
50g apricots
50g cranberries
50g sliced almonds
1 tsp almond extract
500g rolled oats

1. Preheat the oven to 190°C.
2. In a food processor, purée the dates and apple sauce until smooth, then put into a large mixing bowl.
3. Add the bananas and, using a potato masher, mash them into the mixture.
4. Add the apricots, cranberries, sliced almonds and almond extract.
5. Fold in the oats – the mixture should be firm but still moist.
6. Line a 10x6-inch baking pan with parchment paper, add the mixture and smooth out evenly.
7. Bake for 20 minutes, then cool and cut into squares.

## Healthy-ish cocktails

I am quite fond of a drink. I love red wine, but it's full of sugar so I try to avoid it on nights out. I usually stick to vodka with fresh lime and soda when I'm out, but when I have an evening in with the girls, I like to make cocktails.

My go-to cocktails taste really good and are … sort of healthy – well, they would be if I didn't add in the booze, but where's the fun in that?

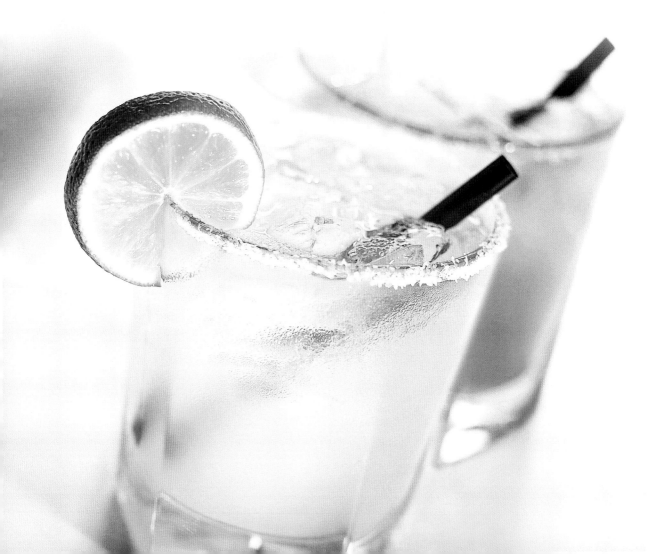

# Classic margarita

35ml tequila

20ml triple sec

10ml freshly squeezed lime juice

flaked rock salt to garnish glass

lime wedge

1. Get a martini glass and add some ice cubes to chill it so it's lovely and cold!
2. Put a layer of the salt on a saucer.
3. Put all spirits together into a shaker with ice and shake the hell out of it for ten seconds.
4. Throw away the ice from the martini glass, rub the rim with the lime wedge and then roll the rim in the saucer of salt.
5. Strain the cocktail mix into the sexy salted glass – and there's a delicious margarita for you!
6. If you want to make it frozen, throw the same ingredients into a blender with a shaker full of ice. Garnish the glass the same way – or if you think salt is not healthy, just garnish with a slice of lime.

# Daquiri delight

This uses natural agave nectar instead of sugar syrup or sugar. Why? 'Cos it's healthy!

50ml rum

20ml lime juice

handful strawberries

handful blackberries

5ml agave nectar

shaker of ice

1. Add all the ingredients to a blender and blitz until smooth and soft.
2. Garnish with extra blackberry and serve in a martini glass.

# Bloody Mary

If you want to make a red snapper instead, replace the vodka with gin. You can use any gin but to make it extra kinky I would add a spiced one – nicey and spicy!

45ml vodka
10ml Worcestershire sauce
3 dashes Tabasco sauce
10ml lemon juice
20ml port
100ml tomato juice
salt and pepper
½ tsp mustard
celery stick to garnish

1.  Stir all the ingredients together in a nice tall glass.
2.  Add the celery stick to garnish and salt and pepper to make it taste sexy!

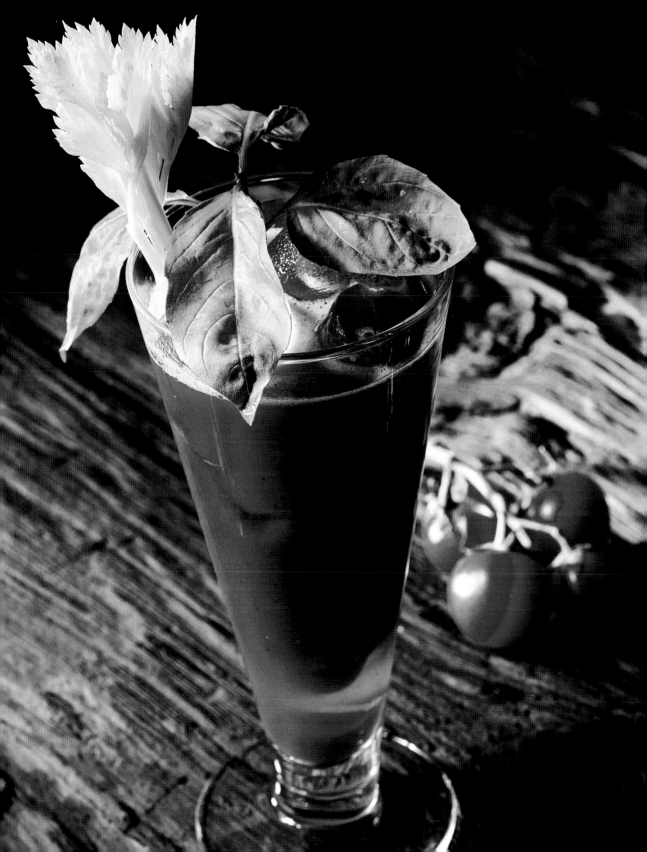

# Mango caprioska

You don't have to use mango for this – you could use strawberries, passion fruit or whatever fruit you like instead.

50ml vodka
3 lime wedges
5ml agave nectar
3 slices mango
crushed ice
soda water

1.  Put limes, mango and agave nectar in a tall glass and muddle together.
2.  Add vodka and stir.
3.  Top with crushed ice, add soda water and garnish with a lime wedge.

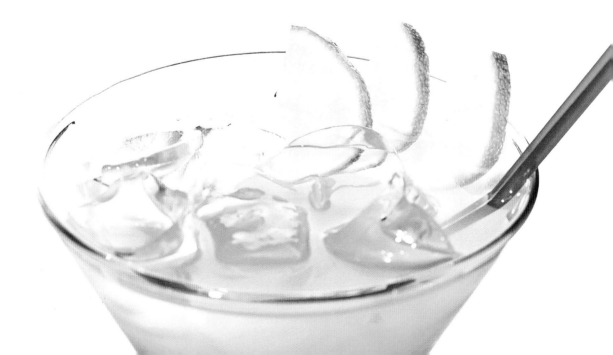

# Hangover help

I thought it was important to follow on from my cocktail recipes with some hangover tips! Now, the obvious thing to do is not get drunk in the first place, but I like a drink and don't plan on giving it up – though I have really cut back on the amount I consume, as too much is just not healthy. Plus I can't afford to have too many hangovers – too much to do! Now, I mostly enjoy alcohol in moderation – a glass of wine with dinner in the evening, for example. But I always like to have my kitchen press stocked with hangover remedies, just in case.

I used to get really bad hangovers, to the point where I couldn't leave the house the day after a night out because of a bad headache or an upset stomach. Now when I'm drinking, I'll have a glass of water every few drinks, which helps a lot.

The day after, I'll usually treat myself to a takeaway – when you're in a delicate state, it's important to be kind to yourself – but I try to order something that will give my body what it needs, like a wood-fired pizza or a pasta dish. A hangover means I'm already massively dehydrated (though drinking water the night before should help), so I usually find it best to avoid salt and any drink other than water.

I have a few things I take religiously for a hangover. I always reach for painkillers for my headache, Dioralyte to help with my dehydration and Berocca to give me a boost of vitamin C. I sometimes also take an anti-nausea tablet if I have a sick tummy.

I don't believe in a 'hair of the dog', as this just makes my hangovers last longer. And while hangover days usually mean a blowout day for me, I do try and drink a green juice at some point, as this always helps. While you're eating treats, it's also good to restore nutrients so the following day you'll be back to yourself!

A shower always makes me feel better and these days I force myself to get up and go out of the house – you always feel worse if you stay on the couch. I suggested a gym session as an option in the previous chapter, but if you don't feel up to this, maybe a trip to the cinema or a coffee with friends will do the trick. It's so easy to stay in bed, but if you get up and about, you'll have earned your nap later.

And that's my final tip – make room for an afternoon nap and, after it, your sore head will be more or less gone!

# My Weekly Food Diary

What I eat varies from week to week, obviously, but this is a food diary for an average week so you can see what's involved. And if anything takes your fancy, you can make it using the recipes included earlier in the chapter. What isn't mentioned below is that I drink lots of water throughout the day – it's so important to keep your body balanced and healthy – and I treat myself to one can of Coke Zero per day (an addiction I refuse to give up).

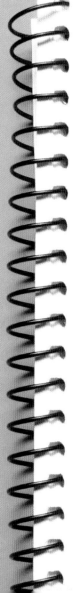

## Monday

Breakfast: two fried eggs on two small pieces of wholegrain toast with half an avocado; two cups of tea

Snack: protein shake

Lunch: wrap with chicken, spinach, tomato and green pesto

Snack: three oat cakes with hummus

Dinner: Thai green curry with a side of boiled rice

Dessert: two squares of dark chocolate
(I try my best to limit it to just two!)

## Tuesday

Breakfast: granola with yoghurt, fresh raspberries and blueberries; two cups of breakfast tea

Snack: protein shake

Lunch: courgetti with arrabiata sauce, topped with Parmesan

Snack: three oat cakes with hummus

Dinner: half a roast chicken with a side of green vegetables and sweet potato wedges

Dessert: Greek yoghurt with blueberries, nuts and agave syrup; a glass of red wine

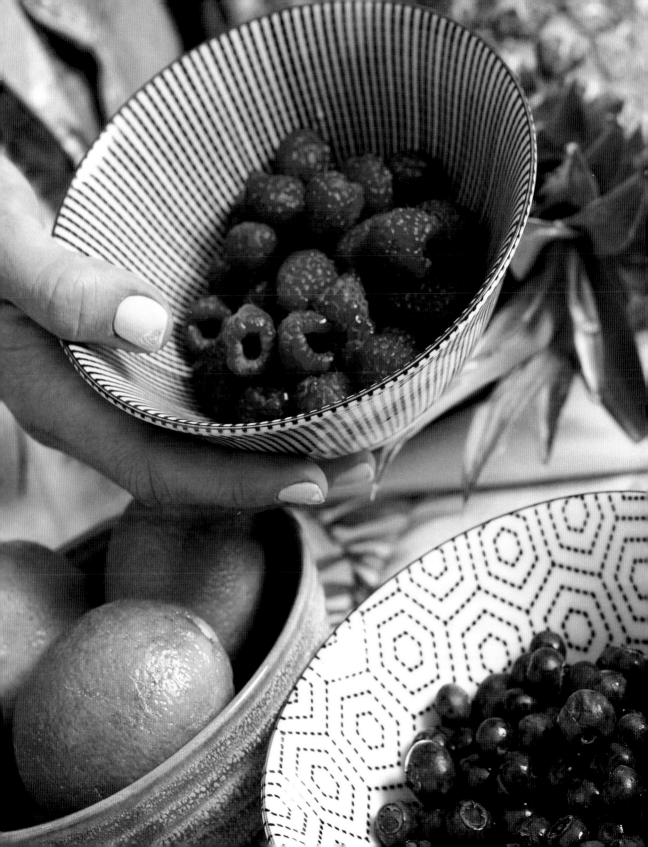

## Wednesday

Breakfast: smoked salmon on brown bread with two poached eggs; two cups of tea

Snack: protein shake

Lunch: Nando's – I love it! They have really great healthy options too.

Snack: none

Dinner: chilli with green beans

Dessert: two squares of dark chocolate

## Thursday

Breakfast: bircher muesli; two cups of tea

Snack: protein shake

Lunch: bulgur salad with chicken

Snack: three oat cakes with hummus

Dinner: fillet steak with spinach and a corn on the cob

Dessert: Greek yoghurt with nuts, blueberries and agave syrup

## Friday

Breakfast: two fried eggs on two small pieces of toast with half an avocado; two cups of tea

Snack: handful of almonds

Lunch: pad-thai at a restaurant

Snack: none

Dinner: leftover bulgur salad with prawns

Dessert: two glasses of red wine (it's the weekend!)

## Saturday and Sunday

At the weekends, I relax on my diet but make sure to keep my all-out, eat-whatever-I- want cheating for one day only, as often I feel sluggish and bloated afterwards – but it makes it easier to steer clear of unhealthy foods in the days that follow. For me, it's the best way to stay on track with a healthy-eating plan for the rest of the time.

# Vitamin and Mineral Supplements

In the past, I was never a fan of taking supplements, but in 2016, my skin became really bad with a bout of adult acne brought on by stress. I decided to look at my diet and see what vitamins and minerals were lacking, and now I use supplements to help make sure I have my recommended daily dose of each one.

Ideally, I would receive all of the nutrients I need from my diet, but it's good to have these supplements to give me a boost. Also, certain nutrients are especially important for women – such as iron (which we can be quite deficient of during our time of the month) and calcium (for healthy bones).

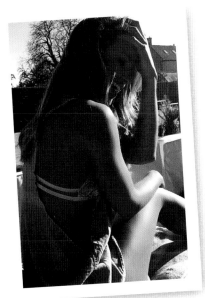

The ones I would recommend to everyone are: vitamin C, magnesium, omega oils and calcium. I have lowered my dairy intake, so I take a supplement to make sure I get all of the calcium I need.

And the ones I take to make up for what's lacking in my diet are: vitamin D, vitamin E and a digestion support. This is because I take medication for acne that is quite harsh on my stomach.

I have to say, I feel so much better for taking them every day. I have noticed the difference in my skin and my overall health after just a few months. Another good thing about them is that I'm pretty sure they've made my hangovers less intense!

*I noticed the difference in my skin and my overall health after just a few months.*

# My top tips for healthy eating

☆ Cook meals in bulk at the start of the week and freeze them, so you always have something nutritious and tasty to eat.

☆ Plan your food shopping carefully. Make a list that matches what meals you plan to batch cook for the week. Make sure you go shopping after you've eaten or you'll be more likely to make bad decisions in the supermarket. And don't buy rubbish – that way it won't be at home to eat when you're having a craving.

☆ Always keep some healthy snacks in your bag or desk at work (my go-to options are fruit, nuts or my protein balls on page 120) – then if you get hungry during the day you have something easily available. If I wait too long between meals, I end up getting really hungry and eat loads of rubbish instead.

☆ When you're ordering a takeaway, go for a healthier option. If I'm ordering an Indian meal, I'll go for a tomato-based sauce and try to stay away from too much naan bread or white rice. I'll order brown rice instead. And go for meals with less sauce – these are usually healthier!

☆ Green juices are a perfect way of adding vegetables to your diet. And supplements are an option for an extra boost of nutrients.

☆ Protein shakes are great for repairing muscle after a workout.

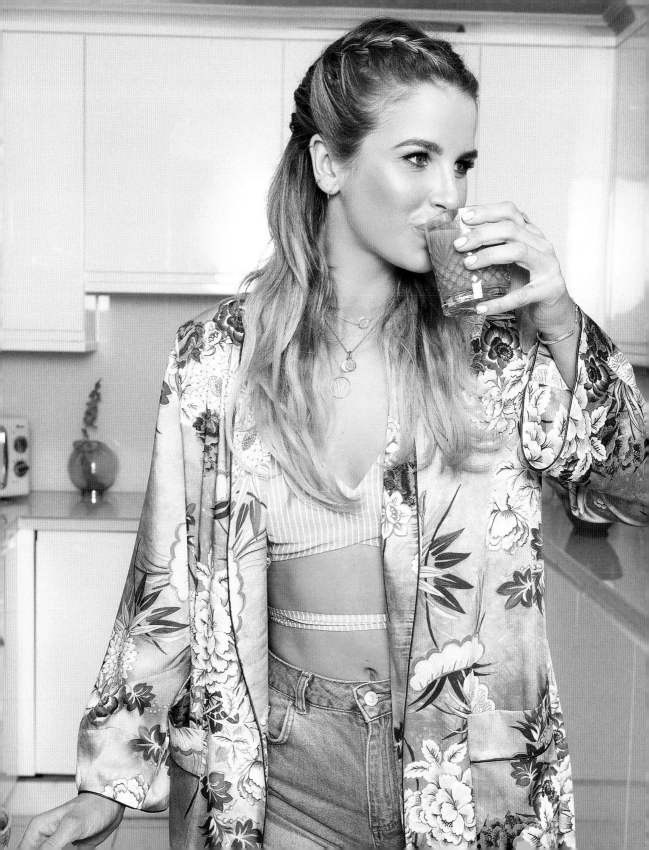

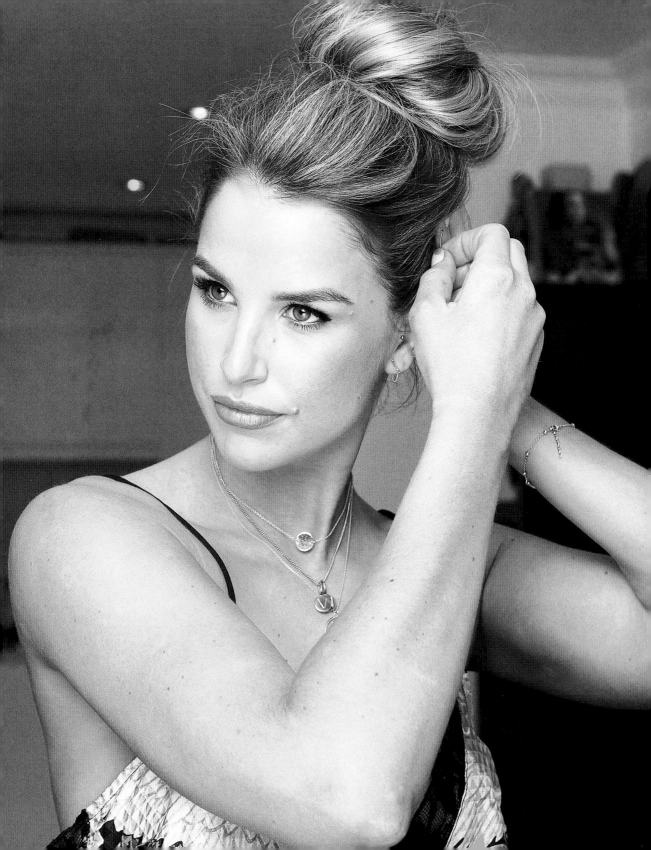

# Beauty

I work in a beauty-focused industry – there are positives and negatives to this, but I definitely don't like to obsess over my appearance too much. There's so much more to people than how they look. But that doesn't mean you can't have fun with it. And, like a lot of women, I love make-up and beauty treatments and getting my nails done. As well as a way of improving or experimenting with how you look, beauty treatments can be a way of treating yourself (I always feel super-relaxed after a facial) and giving your self-confidence a boost.

I do think that people, women especially, are under a lot of pressure to look 'perfect', but this is unattainable – and how boring would life be if we all looked perfect? Social media can add to this pressure quite a bit. I sometimes see comments on my pages from people saying that they would like to have a body like mine, but remember that those pictures are taken from very flattering angles! And photos of me from modelling shoots are often airbrushed, so even I look at them and think, 'Wow, I wish my skin looked like that in real life.' It doesn't.

And I do the same thing. There are so many people I look up to, and when I see their photos on Instagram, I find myself thinking, 'God, I would love to have their body,' but I know I never could because our body types and builds

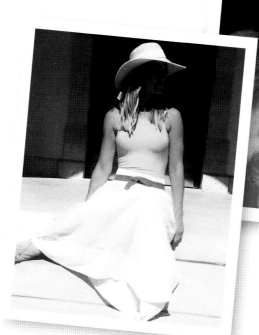

My job allows me to spend a lot of time with experts in the beauty industry and I have learned so many amazing tips and tricks along the way that help me feel more confident.

– and lifestyles – are different. And it's important for me to look at my body in its own right, rather than comparing it to other people's, and to make sure that I'm comfortable in my own skin and feeling good about myself, inside and out.

My job allows me to spend a lot of time with experts in the beauty industry and I have learned so many amazing tips and tricks along the way that help me feel more confident. I keep my beauty regime minimal – I don't think you need to spend a lot of time on yourself to look great, and we are all so time-poor these days that efficiency is key. But there are a couple of things I like to do from time to time to give myself a little extra TLC.

# Skin

## My three essential skincare tips

1. **Water:** I know it sounds boring, but the best thing for your skin, really, is to drink lots of water. I try to drink at least two litres a day.

2. **Cleansing:** It's essential to always remove your make-up properly at the end of the day. Personally, I would never use wipes to remove make-up, as you're basically just rubbing make-up all over your face, and it doesn't take it off very well. If I'm in a rush or it's late after a night out, I use micellar water with cotton pads and then a cleanser to make sure all of the make-up is off.

3. **Sun protection:** I never leave home without having applied a high factor to my face, 30+, even in the winter. My mom has drilled this into me since I was young, although I have only just started wearing it every day – I used to only wear it in the sun. We all have some sun damage on our faces, unless you've worn a mask your entire life, so don't worry about it, but it's sensible to try and limit any future damage.

I've been quite lucky with my skin, until recently it's always been fairly good – but I looked after it really well. That said, in 2016 I got acne for the first time in my life. I know it may seem like I'm over-exaggerating, but it got so bad that some days I didn't want to leave my house. I was surprised by how much it affected my confidence and my sense of self-worth. I found that when I looked in the mirror, all I could see was my bad skin and I became obsessive about it, to an unhealthy degree. In the end, I visited a doctor who prescribed me a six-month course of tablets which really helped to clear it up. As well as the medication, I got a lot of help from my local skin clinic, Renaissance. They gave me advice on what skincare regime would work best for me and I had a lot of different facial treatments that are now getting rid of the red marks the acne left behind.

My skin changes with the seasons – it can be quite oily in the summer and then really dry in the winter – so I always switch up my skincare to match what is happening outside. Here's my daily routine.

# Daily skincare routine

### Morning

I wash my face using a gentle cleanser, making sure that it's not too drying and really cleans my skin. Then I use a serum to hydrate – it also acts as a great make-up primer – and, over that, apply a moisturiser with SPF. I love products from the Image skincare range, especially the Prevention+ daily matte, oil-free moisturiser. My skin feels hydrated without looking oily. Then I apply my make-up, if needed!

I'm a big fan of Crème de la Mer products too – they have a brilliant micellar water that I sometimes use in the mornings, followed by their moisturiser.

### Night-time

I love the Bioderma micellar water, which I sometimes use to take my make-up off at night – it works really well at getting rid of any traces of make-up. Afterwards, I'll cleanse my face and then apply a serum, followed by moisturiser. The Body Shop do amazing oils and moisturisers that I use too when I need to switch up my skincare regime – I'm a big fan of their Vitamin E range.

## Weekly Routine

### My at-home facial

I don't always have time to go to a salon for a facial, so sometimes I just do a quick one at home. It's easy and your skin will feel amazing after it.

I do this at-home facial once a week, and I always use an exfoliator with a small amount of glycolic acid in it – my favourite is Benefit's Refined Finish Facial Polish, which is very gentle on my skin. Glycolic acid is great for treating fine lines, acne, blackheads, dullness and oiliness.

**Step 1:** Make sure your face is completely make-up free – cleanse your skin to remove any impurities.

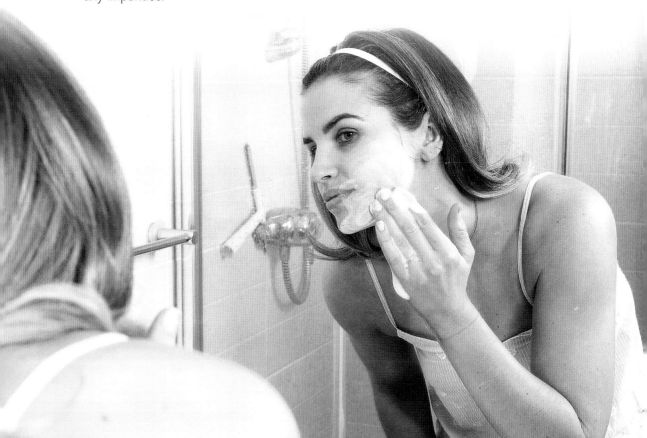

**Step 2:** Steam time! Steaming your face is a great way to open your pores so you can clean them out. I don't have a steam machine, so I put hot water in a bowl, put my face over it and cover my head with a towel. You can also put a face cloth in warm water and then place it over your face to achieve the same effect. You need to do this a few times so it gets a good steaming.

**Step 3:** Next, exfoliate your skin. Your pores will be open so exfoliating will clean out all those unwanted blackheads. Then wash your face with water to remove the exfoliator.

**Step 4:** Apply your face mask. I like a clay one like the Glamglow from Boots and the Charlotte Tilbury clay mask, which is expensive, but I sometimes make my own. Leave the face mask on for fifteen to twenty minutes – this is a good opportunity to take some time for yourself.

**Step 5:** When you have washed off your face mask, you need to apply a thick moisturiser. Everyone has their favourite, but I like to go with one that is perfume-free and, again, usually from my favourite range from Image.

## Avocado face-mask recipe

Avocado is not only great for your body – it's brilliant for your skin too. As well as eating it every day, I love using it in face masks, as the antioxidants are good for glowing skin and help with anti-ageing.

½ avocado
big spoon of honey

1. Scoop the avocado flesh into a bowl.
2. Mash until it is smooth.
3. Add the honey and mix it all together.
4. Apply to your face and leave it on for fifteen to twenty minutes before rinsing.

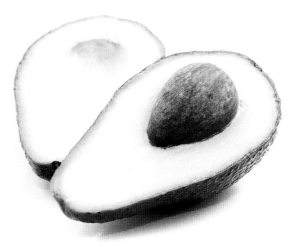

# Skincare for different skin types

No two people need the exact same thing when it comes to their skin, and you need to ensure that you use products suited to what your skin needs. So I had a chat with Kristina Kelly from Renaissance Clinic in Howth to get some advice on how to look after the most common skin types and problems.

## Dry, sensitive, rosacea skin

Use products that contain vitamin C, which is an antioxidant and protects the skin from free-radical damage. Applying it to your skin is more effective than taking a supplement or getting the vitamin from your food. It will soothe, nourish and hydrate your skin, and also accelerate collagen synthesis.

**Products recommended:** The Vital C range from Image Skincare, especially Vital C Hydrating Anti-Aging Serum which can be used morning and evening after you have cleansed your skin but before you apply moisturiser. This will rejuvenate dull, dry and tired skin. The Renaissance Clinic stock the Image range which I love but I also find Nivea Crème a brilliant budget-friendly moisturiser.

## Oily, acne-prone skin

Use oil-free products that contain a BHA, such as salicylic acid. This will remove surface oil and bacteria and help reduce the production of oil. If there is a lot of congestion, an AHA is also needed, which is glycolic acid. This will help exfoliate and resurface your skin.

**Products recommended:** Clear Cell range and Ageless range from Image skincare.

> ☆ **Top tip:** If you have very active/live acne, stay clear of grainy exfoliators, as they will only spread bacteria and cause further spots.

## Combination/unbalanced skin

If you are a teenager, pregnant or male, or if your skin is unbalanced, you need products that are going to soothe, heal and hydrate the skin. I would always suggest getting a skin facial analysis, especially if your skin is problematic, so you know exactly what you should be using for it.

**Products recommended:** Ormedic, Iluma and Prevention+ range from Image skincare.

## Dehydrated skin

This is often confused with dry skin, but whereas dry skin is caused by a lack of oil, dehydrated skin is a lack of water. Dehydrated skin will feel tight directly after washing your face. I always try to drink at least two litres of water a day, but even with that I still get dehydrated skin.

If I am having a bad skin day, I apply a moisture mask for about twenty minutes at night. I then put face oil and moisturising cream on over it. Dehydrated skin can be a nightmare – especially when you wear make-up, as it can catch in it. I also take Omega 3, 6 and 9 supplements that help lock moisture into your skin.

**Products recommended:** I have a ton of masks I love using, but my number one is definitely the Charlotte Tilbury mud mask – it will make your skin feel amazing. I use some sort of mask at least once a week.

# Anti-ageing

There are so many anti-ageing products on the market, some of which I started using when I was about twenty-two – it's all about prevention, so it's good to start young.

I change up my skincare quite a lot, so I know a lot of the anti-ageing products do work. A facial a month is also a great way to get good anti-ageing results without having to go down the Botox route. I love the Max range in Image Skincare – it's nicknamed 'Botox in a bottle'! And I'm a big fan of the Protect & Perfect range from No7.

I'm often asked whether I would consider surgery or Botox or fillers and, quite simply,

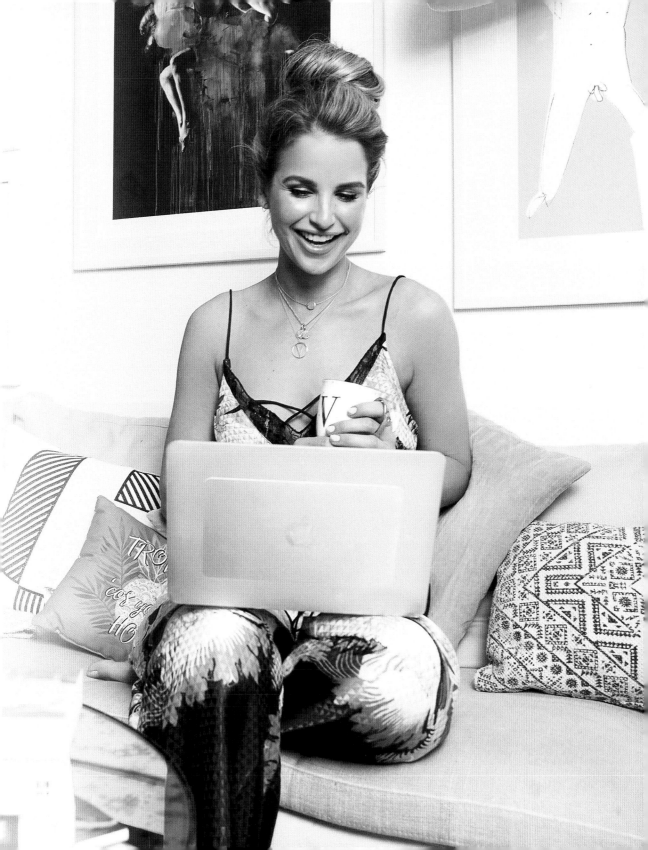

the answer is yes. I don't think I would go down the surgery route, but with all of the amazing treatments available these days, I don't think I'll have a need for it. The thought of a facelift scares me at any age – and I don't like the idea of ending up with a face that couldn't express the full extent of my emotions or left me looking less like myself.

## Vitamin A: The best-kept secret!

Dermatologists, plastic surgeons and beauticians all over the world agree: vitamin A is an essential ingredient in guaranteeing long-term skin health. Vitamin A is simply a game-changer for healthy skin and is the king of anti-ageing.

Vitamin A repairs at a cellular level, acts as a natural exfoliant, promotes skin health, assists the repair of pigmentation, brings clarity, plumps up the epidermis (the skin's top layer), stimulates collagen and increases internal moisture levels.

A good vitamin A serum will:

* deliver pure active ingredients
* ensure fast delivery into the skin's deeper layers
* not cause irritation
* have long-lasting results

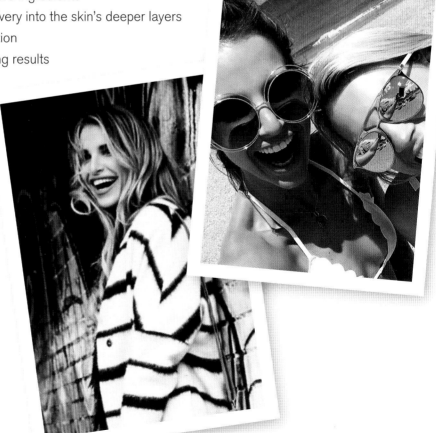

A facelift scares me. I don't like the idea of ending up with a face that couldn't express the full extent of my emotions.

My go-to vitamin A products are, once again, from Image. And I love Obaji products – they have a brilliant Vitamin A serum.

## My favourite facials

I'm a huge fan of all beauty treatments and, in particular, any treatment that can make my skin look better. I love having facials – they are a great way to relax and improve your skin. I try to have one at least once a month to treat my skin and make sure it's getting the love it deserves.

Because I have a beauty section on my blog, I get invited to try a lot of different facials, so I have included the ones that worked best for me. These are available at most salons, though do be careful to go to a recommended one!

### Collagen wave

One of my favourite facials is a collagen wave. It's an anti-ageing facial and is more about prevention of lines and wrinkles – it's important to start thinking about anti-ageing once you reach your mid-twenties (slightly depressing, I know!). I used to have one of these facials on a monthly basis but now I get them every few months.

A collagen wave facial involves blasting your skin with radio frequency waves to encourage collagen production, which is what makes us look young. The first step is to have your skin analysed and cleansed, after which a nourishing petite serum is added. A gel is applied to the machine, which looks like a curling tong, so it can glide easily over your face. The tong heats the skin's layers to forty degrees, which is the temperature needed for the skin to produce more collagen, and then radio frequency waves are transmitted onto the skin.

The procedure lasts between forty-five minutes and an hour, and then the gel is removed and a soothing mask is applied. Your face will be slightly red after this treatment, but it goes away when your skin cools down. I have had this facial at least fifty times and it definitely works.

## Skin peels

After my recent bad bout of acne I had some scarring, which I have been treating with skin peels in the Renaissance Clinic. I had three peels and then moved on to derma rolling, which is a little more invasive but great for helping with scarring and rejuvenating skin. Derma rolling creates tiny punctures in the skin to stimulate tissue repair. I did need two days' downtime afterwards, as I was left a bit red and swollen, but the results were definitely worth it and my skin is almost back to the way it was.

Skin peels sound so much worse than they really are – the sight of Samantha from *Sex and the City* after her peel would put anyone off, but, I promise, you won't look like her after one!

During the treatment, a chemical is applied to remove the top layer of your skin, so your skin will be a little bit flaky for a few days, but when this goes away, your skin will look really nice and clear.

I was told that as you get older your skin doesn't shed the dead top skin as easily, so that's the reason peels are so good. I had my first peel three years ago and I love how it makes my skin look. And though you do need a few days' downtime after them too, I have gone out with my flaky skin, and it only looks bad if you look really closely.

## Collagen induction therapy

Collagen induction therapy (CIT), also known as 'micro-needling', is an aesthetic medical procedure that involves repeatedly puncturing the skin with tiny sterile needles to induce endogenous production of collagen. It is an effective treatment for acne scars, skin rejuvenation, fine lines and wrinkles.

I wouldn't say it's the most comfortable treatment I've ever had, but the pain was bearable and I will be getting it done again. My face was quite red afterwards and fairly

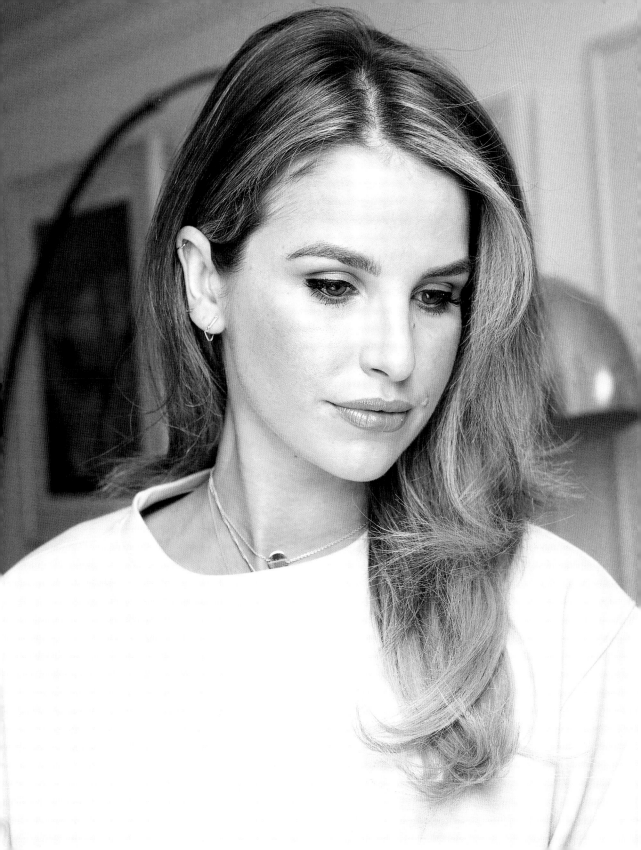

dry and tight. The day after the treatment, my face wasn't nearly as red but was a little dry and scratched. I looked after it by applying plenty of moisturiser and staying out of the sun. By day three, I was wearing make-up again and was, for the most part, back to normal. I could already notice a difference in my skin but the best results came a couple of weeks later. I have to say I really loved this treatment – I obviously hated the first two days but, now, the scarring is almost invisible.

### The vampire facial

The vampire facial is a bizarre concept, but after I'd seen it on TV I wanted to give it a try. In terms of invasiveness, this is the furthest I have gone with a treatment. The results, though, are unbelievable and last up to nine months. I noticed a difference in my skin a couple of weeks after the treatment and this has continued as the treatment carries on working, so I think I will be going for this one again.

Blood is taken from your arm to fill four vials that are then spun in a centrifuge for ten minutes. This separates your blood into layers of blood, stem cells and plasma. After this comes the more painful bit, although I was laughing while getting it done, so it wasn't too bad (and I have a very low pain threshold!).

Your face is numbed with a cream and then a needle is put into the area being treated to make a small hole, which isn't noticeable. After they put the needle in, they move it around while injecting the plasma back into your face. I had it done in three areas of my face and had a little bit of swelling the next day, but it was unnoticeable to other people. The plasma naturally rushes to places that need restoring, and areas that have lost elasticity or collagen will get it first. I know it sounds a bit drastic, but it's like a natural form of Botox, as it's all from your own body.

# Holiday skin

Any break from our normal routines can make keeping up our good habits when it comes to skincare quite tricky – and a holiday means that our skin requirements might change. So I thought I would add some tips about looking after your skin when you go away, especially if you're going on a sun holiday.

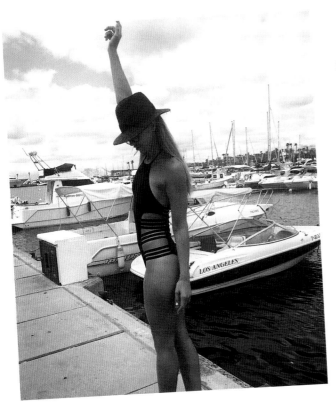

A flight dehydrates your skin, even if it's only a short one. Because of this, I never drink alcohol on a flight – I stick to water. If I'm on a long-haul flight, I always bring a cleanser to take off my make-up and then apply a good moisturiser during the flight.

Although the sun is harmful to your skin if it's not protected by sunscreen, it is good for your overall health and is our main source of vitamin D. We all feel better in the sun and it's not just because it's lovely and warm. Sunlight is related to the production of serotonin neurotransmitters, which make us feel happy. The problem with exposure to the sun is when people spend excessive amounts of time in it without using sunscreen – they end up looking more like a roasted lobster by the end of the day and expose themselves to dangerous UV rays, which cause serious long-term damage to skin and increase the risk of skin cancer. The level of SPF you use is very important. I tan quite easily but always use factor 50 on my face, neck, hands and chest and factor 20 for the rest of my body. I reapply every couple of hours or after being in the water.

I did spend some of my youth with baby oil on my legs and arms but I would never ever do that again – it totally ruins your skin.

Your face is the part of your body that gets the worst sun damage so even in winter you should wear an SPF. In the sun, I always wear a hat to cover my face too.

*I always wear a hat to cover my face in the sun.*

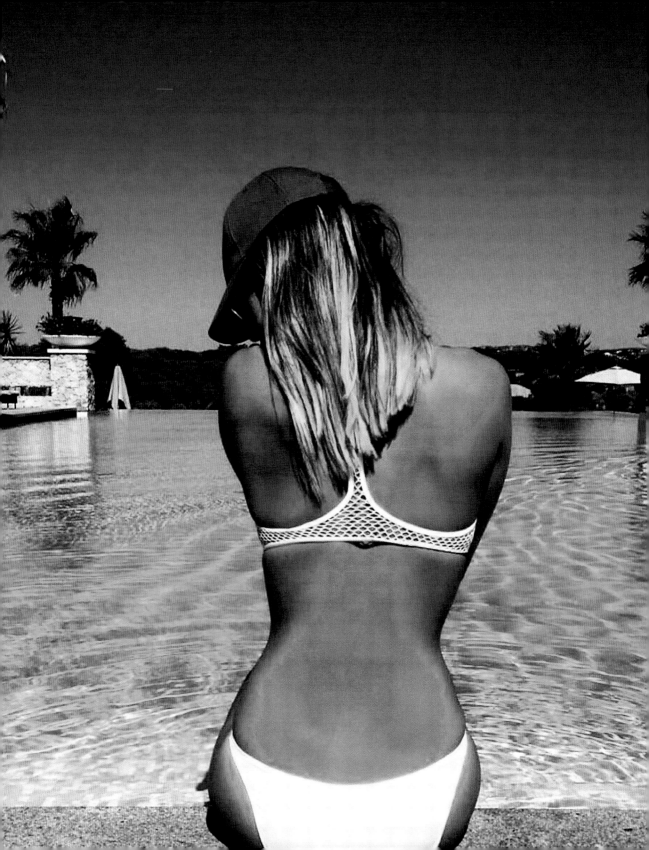

# Body

## Moisturising

My all-time favourite body moisturiser is Bioderma – they often have great deals on this in the airport. My mom always gives me a bottle for birthdays and Christmas, it smells amazing and it's really good on your skin. I *always* moisturise my whole body after a shower – I feel my skin getting dry if I don't. I don't like really thick body moisturisers, as I feel they stick to my skin and make it feel clammy.

## Tanning tips

I always wear fake tan – it makes me feel and look better. Over the years, I have experienced a million fake-tan horror stories (orange hands were my signature look in secondary school), but since then I have fronted some tanning campaigns so I have learned quite a few tips to get the perfect glow.

It may be annoying, but you *always* have to exfoliate before a tanning session. I put on my exfoliator gloves and use a good body exfoliator to scrub my skin. You may need to do this a couple of days in advance if you are trying to remove a previous tan. I love the Body Shop exfoliator, as it makes your skin feel really smooth, but really I could use any product on the shelf – I have yet to come across a bad exfoliator.

I then dry my skin and rub a good bit of moisturiser on my elbows, knees, feet and hands. It makes the product go on these tricky areas much better. But it's best not to moisturise your body all over, as it can make the tan slippy and it won't take to your skin properly. Even when I go for a spray, I put it on these parts.

I don't always use a mitt when I apply tan – it depends on the product I'm using. If I don't use a mitt, I make sure to wash my hands as soon as I have finished. I then put a little product on one hand but have to use a mitt to rub this part in, paying extra attention to my wrists so the tan blends properly, then I do my other hand.

Always wear dark, loose clothes after applying a tan – you don't want anything tight as it will mark the tan, and anything light will get stained. I leave my tan on overnight and then wash it off in the morning.

Make sure to moisturise every day when you have a tan on, as it keeps it even and it comes off without looking like you have something wrong with your skin.

There are so many self-tanning products on the market, from creams to mousses to sprays. What you should be aiming for is a relatively natural look – the colour your skin would be after a two- or three-week sun holiday. My favourite ones are St. Tropez, Sunkiss, Bellamianta and James Read – they all look natural and last for ages.

# Nails, Nails, Nails

Is it just me, or do you feel so much better when your nails are done?

I wear different colours for different seasons, although I think you can wear a fire-engine red any time of year. In the summer, I go mad for neons – I love the pop of colour – or else I do a nude or all-over white, which is probably my favourite. In the winter, I stick with reds, nudes and darker colours to match the darker-coloured clothes I tend to wear at that time of year.

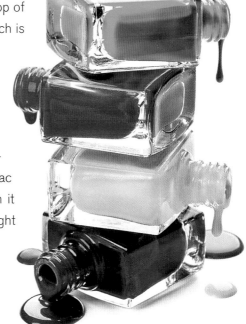

Some colours don't suit certain skin tones, so try on a little polish before deciding on a colour – this is especially important if you're opting for shellac or Gelish because otherwise you'll be stuck with it for two weeks. I have a yellowish skin tone, so light yellows and blues don't look good on me at all.

I love getting my nails done – I feel that it completes an outfit and allows you to dip your toe in the water when it comes to having fun with colour and design. I usually opt for shellac or Gelish, as it lasts so much longer and I don't have to worry much about it chipping.

I asked Andrea Horan, who owns funky Dublin nail salon Tropical Popical, for advice on how to keep your manicure at its best.

## Tropical Popical's top tips for maintaining your manicure

- ✫ Never pull or pick your gel polish or extensions off. You're also pulling the top layer of your nail. *Gross!* You should have your gel polish/extensions removed properly at a salon.

- ✫ Use cuticle oil every day. Keep it beside your toothbrush so that every time you brush your teeth you remember to apply some oil.

- ✫ Use rubber gloves for any cleaning, washing up or gardening. Personally, we try to avoid cleaning at all costs, but maybe that's just us.

- ✫ Don't leave your hands soaking in a gorge bubbling hot bath or spend your time hanging around saunas or steam rooms.

- ✫ Don't cut or file your nails when you have a gel polish on (what the hell do you think we're here for?) as it gets rid of the seal.

- ✫ Simple things like peeling stickers from magazines or opening cans can break the seal so be super careful (or better yet, get someone else to do it for you).

- ✫ When you're living the actual tropical life, make sure to wipe sunscreen, chlorine and insect repellent off your gel polish as it can stain (fake tan can too).

☆ Get a full manicure before your first set of gel extensions and then after every two to four sets. If any cuticle is left on the nail, the gel can't bond properly. Also, the closer the gel can get to the cuticle, the longer your gels will last.

☆ Use non-acetone nail polish remover and base coat when changing polish on gel extensions.

☆ Hand creams that contain lanolin can cause lifting.

☆ Gels need to be refilled every two and a half to three and a half weeks.

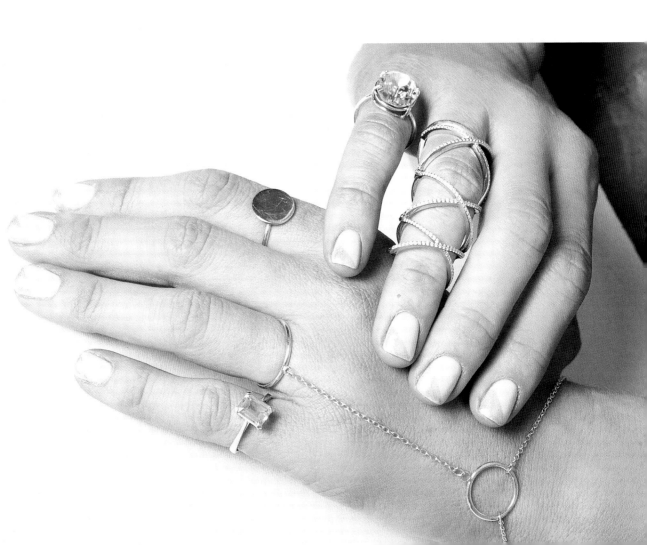

★ You should get a full file off and new tips etc. every three to four refills to make sure the new gel is touching the nail and all the old gel that might have been lifting is gone. It should never be a continuous cycle of refills.

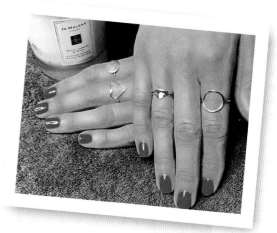

*I wear different colours for different seasons, although I think you can wear a fire-engine red any time of year.*

# Face

## Eyebrows

Eyebrows are one of the most important features on your face and can totally change the way you look.

I think many of us plucked our brows to within an inch of their lives when we were younger – not a good look! Today, I think most of us strive for a thicker brow – thankfully, because the upkeep is much easier.

I only started getting my brows done by a professional around three years ago, and now I can't go without having them done every couple of months by a HD brow artist. Then I just pluck the regrowth myself, keeping to the shape that was created for me. I also stick to this shape when I fill in my brows and never go overboard – you want your brows to look full, but not drawn on.

I was on a dancing show the first time I had my brows done – I had decided to try a blade-type trimmer myself, which is a small blade that trims the eyebrow, but I took too much off and the results were disastrous. Luck was on my side because backstage, doing facials and brows, was Nilam Patel, co-founder of beauty brand High Definition. During my time on the show, she transformed my brows and I love them now.

I decided that, to get the best advice on eyebrows, I should go straight to the professional, so the sections below are Nilam's pearls of wisdom when it comes to brows.

* Your eyebrows create a frame for your eyes and face. The right brow shape can make your face look slimmer, your nose look smaller and your eyes look bigger, so getting this right is really important.

* Have your brows done professionally, even if it is just once, to get your ideal shape and to get you on track. Your brows should complement your skin and hair colouring, your personality and your personal style. Your stylist should advise you on your ideal shape, and if you don't have enough hair when you have them done, you should try to grow them into that shape over time.

* Remember, no two brows are exactly the same because we have different hair growth, bone structure and fatty tissue on each side of our faces – 'brows are sisters not twins'. If you struggle with symmetry, at least ensure your brows are friends.

There is no single perfect brow style that suits everyone. Your brows should be as individual to you as your fingerprints. The ideal size, colour, shape and angle will vary from person to person. Saying that, everyone can create their perfect brow by following these guidelines.

## The right colour

Ensure you match your brow colour to your hair and skin tone.

* If you have warm skin and hair, go with a warm colour (orangey-red undertone) and cool skin tones should go for cooler colours (ashy undertone).

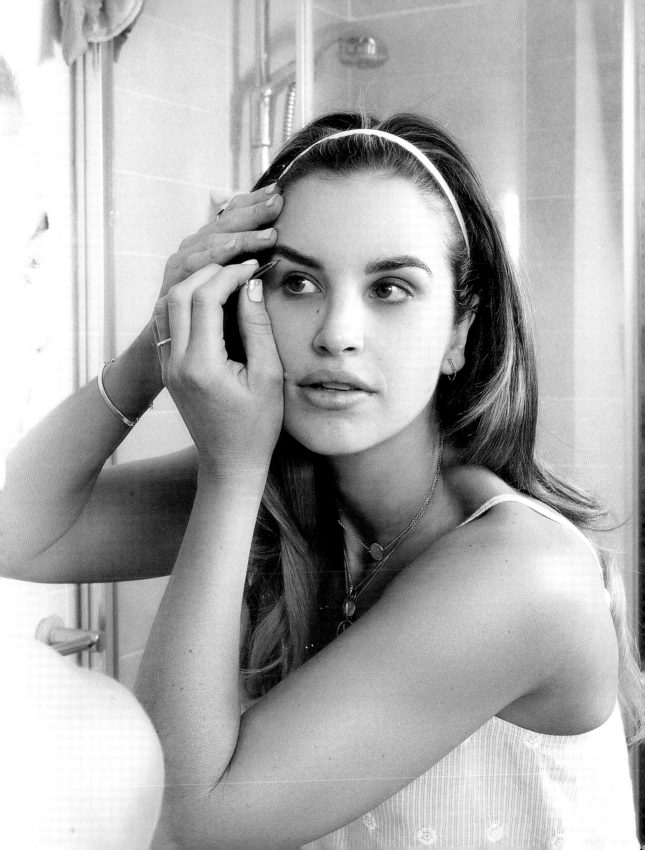

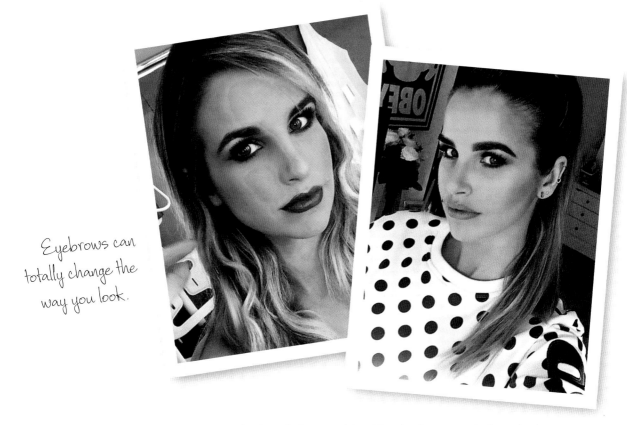

*Eyebrows can totally change the way you look.*

* When it comes to depth of colour, I always advise blondes to go one to two shades darker than their hair colour, and those with darker hair to go one to two shades lighter.

* Redheads should stick to a similar depth of colour to their hair.

* Pastel/white or grey hair should aim to go extremely fair and ashy.

## The right size and position

Getting the size or position of the brow wrong can make or break your look. If your brows are too high, you will look surprised; if they are too low, you will look moody. If you pick the fatty tissue that sits on your brow bone, the eyebrow should sit between your fingers. If you have a small face, avoid a brow that is too heavy. Your brows should not dominate your face. If you have a large face, avoid a thin brow as your face and features will look larger.

## The right shape and angles

Make sure your brows look natural for your face. You can always exaggerate and temporarily alter the shape with make-up. Your brows should follow a slight incline from bulb to arch and a slight decline from arch to tail.

* If you have an angular face shape and features, stick to squarer, more angled brows.

* If you have rounder features, keep some soft curves in the brow shape.

* If you have a long face, then keep your brows flatter, as an arch will lengthen the face more.

* If you have a short face, then try to lift the arch, as this will make the face look longer.

* A wide nose can be made to look slimmer by keeping the brows closer together and the opposite works for a long, thin nose.

## Over-plucking

This is a big no-no, but it is so common. Unless you are blessed with bushy eyebrows, trying to pluck your way to symmetry is only going to lead to skinny, misshapen brows. It's OK to have some fluffy hairs, so don't use a magnifying mirror that makes each hair look gigantic, and swap from brow to brow rather than finishing one completely and trying to match the other.

## Never shave your brows

One slip and it could all be over!

## From the top

Contrary to myth, tidying the top can help create symmetry and prevent brows looking too high and surprised.

### Tweezing your own brows

If you must do your own brows, then follow these tips to make sure you don't end up with 'barely there' brows.

* Using an eyebrow pencil, draw them into the shape you want, making sure you can still see all the hairs.

* Remember, you may have to 'cheat' the perfect shape with make-up to make them look fuller and more symmetrical, so don't be afraid to draw outside your natural hair growth (within reason) or to leave some hairs to grow in.

* When you have the desired shape, trim any long, unruly hairs first, one by one.

* Tweeze only the stray hairs around the shape.

☆ **Top tip:** Given the right care, even the most over-plucked brows can grow back into a better shape. If you had a fairly full brow when you were a teen, they should grow back. The longer brows are over-plucked and the older you are, the slower the regrowth will be. But persevere because brows really can change your whole face.

## Lashes

I love using false lashes when I'm going out, but I like to keep them as natural as possible – it's the same approach I have with my make-up – I don't like looking overdone.

I think false lashes open up your eyes and are essential if you're feeling (or looking) tired – you know, one of those days when your eyes look constantly half shut. I call it 'newborn-baby eyes' and it's not a good look for a grown adult!

When I wear false lashes, I wear individual ones, as they look more natural and are

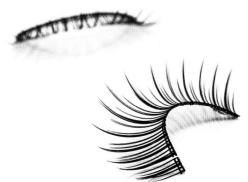

really easy to use. I like to use the short ones, which are still longer than my own lashes, so that I can build up a good volume. I like Penneys individuals but I also love the Eylure and Ardell ones.

I like to do my eye make-up before applying lashes. Then I put some of the glue – it's important to use a good one that dries clear – on the back on my hand and leave it for a couple of minutes. Next, I use tweezers to pick up an individual lash – tweezers make it a lot easier to place the lashes in the right position on my lash line. I put the tip of the lash in the glue and leave it to dry a little before placing it.

Then I keep applying lashes until I'm happy with the finished look. I add an extra bit of eyeliner when the glue has dried and put some mascara on the lashes.

I have had permanent lashes before and, as with hair extensions, they can be quite addictive! Permanent lashes can make you look better when you have no make-up on, and make-up effort is minimal because the lashes also create a slight liner effect on your top lid. They last at least a month and I definitely don't stick to the rules with these! I wear mascara and I am quite rough with them – though they'll last longer if you are nice to them!

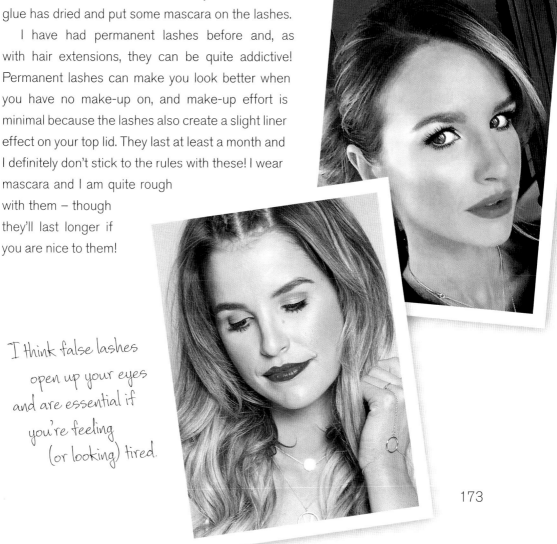

I think false lashes open up your eyes and are essential if you're feeling (or looking) tired.

173

# Make-up

I get my make-up done for work a lot, and I love it – it's such a creative process, and make-up artists are constantly trying out looks on my face that I never would have considered, let alone attempted. I always pay close attention so I can give it a go myself at home. My go-to make-up look is one I call 'daytime smoky' – dark eye make-up, though not too heavy, with a nude lip. But I like to change it up, depending on my mood – a pop of colour on my lips for a party or a natural bronzed look for summertime.

Although I'm pretty good at doing my own make-up, I wanted to get tips from a couple of professionals so I asked Ashley O'Rourke, a make-up artist I've known for ten years, for her top tips. Ashley's speciality is gorgeous-looking skin – she can transform your face while still making sure you look like yourself. I also spoke to another amazing make-up artist named Rebecca Todd, who has created a few looks for me. Along with a step-by-step guide to each look, I'll include a full product list of what was used. Of course, you can adapt it to what products you have in your make-up bag, but I know that I'm always on the lookout for recommendations so I wanted to share mine with you.

I'm also going to give you a couple of step-by-step guides to my own go-to make-up looks. I don't like make-up that is too heavy – I like to look like myself, just a slightly more polished version. But first, a look inside my make-up bag …

## My make-up bag

My make-up bag is pretty massive – my job means that I'm being introduced to new looks and new products all the time, and I'm very keen to try them all! But as I travel a lot, I have to be ruthless and scale this down to the essentials – and because I have some tried-and-tested looks that I use all the time, I know exactly what I need in my bag to achieve these. Here are the products I can't live without.

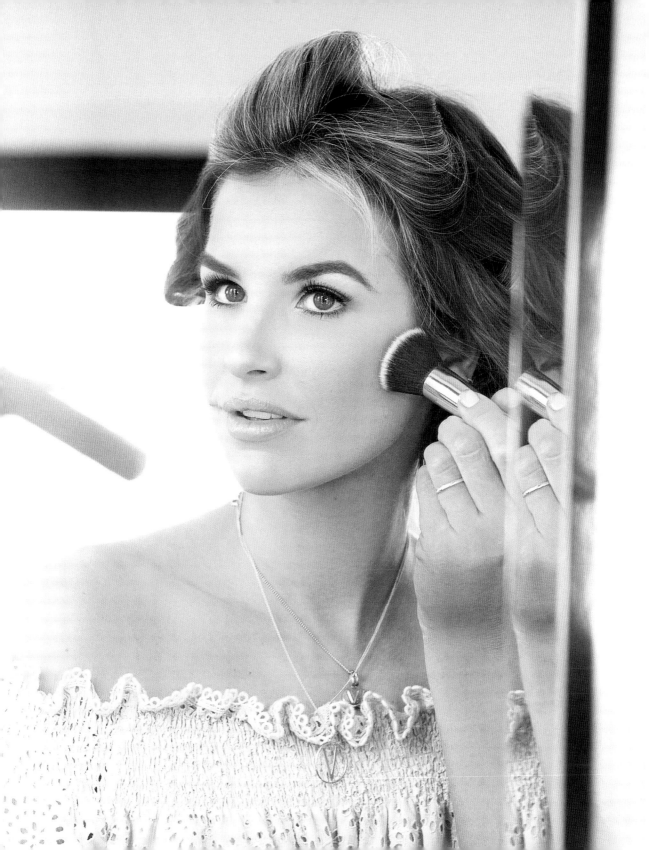

## Brushes

These are a staple of any make-up bag and, because they get so much use, it's important to make sure you have a good set. I currently use brushes from the Callanberry range, which I adore. These were a bit of a splurge (though well worth it!), but if you're looking for a fantastic set of brushes at a more affordable price, I would go for the Real Techniques range, which is available in Boots and other pharmacies. You might want to build up your brush collection slowly rather than investing in a complete set, so here are the key tools you'll want in your kit: foundation brush, bronzer/contour brush, eyeshadow brush, blusher brush (if you use a powder product) and eyeliner brush. And do make sure you look after your brushes, especially if you've invested a lot of money in them – they should be cleaned regularly.

## Cleaning your brushes

☆ Fill a bowl with warm water – not too hot.

☆ Immerse your brushes in the water – only the hairs and not above the handle, as you don't want the hairs becoming loose.

☆ Squirt a mild detergent onto the palm of your hand. I normally use baby shampoo, as it's mild but foamy enough for washing.

☆ Then wash the brush hairs in the shampoo, creating a good lather. Do this for four or five minutes to make sure all traces of make-up and any bacteria and dirt are caught up in the soap.

★  Rinse brushes carefully in a fresh bowl of water.

★  To make sure they are squeaky clean, I normally rinse the tips of the brushes under a warm tap afterwards too.

★  Lay on a towel to dry.

## Highlighter

I always use a liquid highlighter under my foundation to create a dewy make-up look. It is quite muted once you apply your foundation but it will make your skin look gorgeous. TheBalm Mary-Lou Manizer is one I use regularly.

## Primer

If I am having a bad week with my skin, I always use Benefit Porefessional. It smoothes the skin and helps cover any blemishes before you apply foundation.

## Foundation

The key to foundation is to get the perfect match for your skin type and tone. I have been through a million foundations and still change mine when I finish a bottle, as I feel like my skin gets used to a certain one and then after a while it doesn't work as well.

I don't like a heavy foundation – I think if you use one that is heavy, it can make you look older and you don't want to completely block out your skin. I use a light foundation that I build up in the areas that need it most. At the moment I'm using Charlotte Tilbury, Nars and HD foundations.

## Concealer

This would be on my desert-island list – I cannot live without concealer. I have dark circles under my eyes, which can be the result of not drinking enough water or getting enough sleep, but I've had them my whole life. They don't bother me too much, but I do cover them with concealer. I personally love the lift concealer from Make Up For Ever and Nars have a brilliant one too.

I also have a concealer trio from Make Up For Ever containing three different shades that I use under my eyes, on my eyelids and on my nose to even out the colour of my skin. And when it comes to covering up blemishes, I love Charlotte Tilbury's The Retoucher. It's a really light concealer but gives good coverage.

## Powder

A powder over your foundation will keep your make-up in place for a lot longer. I use both a pressed and a loose powder, but always in a neutral shade. I don't add powder for coverage or colour, just to ensure that my make-up is set. I love the Charlotte Tilbury pressed powder, and Banana Powder is a loose powder which loads of make-up artists use.

## Blusher

I think blusher is the finishing touch. It wakes your face up and gives you a healthy glow. I switch colours in my blusher all the time, but my favourite is a soft pink. We all have different colouring, so it's best to go to a make-up counter and ask for help finding the perfect blusher for your skin type.

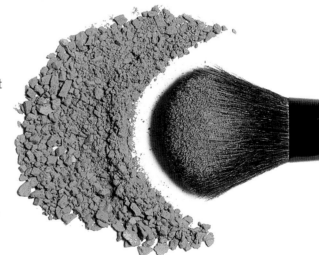

## Powder highlighter

It's nice for your skin to glow a little, and I achieve this by using a powder highlighter and the liquid one before foundation. There are lots of types out there, but I like a gold one. I use it across my cheekbones, down the front of my nose, on my cupid's bow, the corner of my eyes and on my brow bone. This will reflect any light and make your skin look glowing – don't go too overboard with it, though, or you'll just look shiny, which isn't a good look!

## Lips

A good lip – red, nude or a strong burgundy – can make an outfit. Before I begin my make-up, I make sure my lips are prepped. It's best to make sure your lips are as soft as possible, especially if you're planning to wear a matte shade.

I like to apply a lip balm or a primer (such as the MAC Prep + Prime Lip) to get my lips as soft as possible, which helps the lipstick to sit better – but you don't want them too slippy, so blot off any excess with a tissue. After this, I'll apply lip liner and lipstick – using the techniques mentioned on page 187. Lip liner is an essential tool – using it makes your lips more defined, helps your lip colour stay on longer and can even make your lips look fuller (more on this shortly). Sometimes I don't even bother with lipstick or gloss – I'll fill in my lips using the lip liner and then add some lip balm on top. I'm a big fan of the Charlotte Tilbury lip liner range.

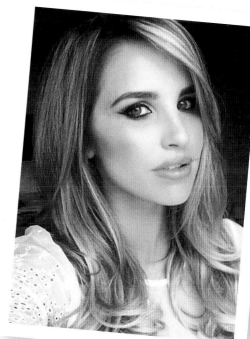

## Eyeliner

I wear eyeliner every day on my top lids. My eyes aren't huge, so this definitely helps to open them up and make them look bigger. I usually use a L'Oréal liquid liner – it's super easy to apply and lasts all day. If I want a more dramatic eyeliner, I use a gel liner that I apply with a brush. My go-to liner is MAC Fluidline in black but I sometimes change it up by wearing brown or purple.

*When I want dramatic eyeliner I use a gel liner that I apply with a brush.*

### Mascara

A look is never finished without mascara. I always go for a volumising one because I like a strong focus on my eyes when it comes to make-up. I've found that you don't need to splash out on mascara to find a good one – there are lots of fantastic budget-friendly products out there. My picks are Maybelline and Benefit, but for an expensive option I adore the YSL one.

### Body shimmer

Body shimmer is great for giving you slimmer-looking legs, and I always use it when I wear anything where my legs are on show. I rub it down the front and backs of my legs and it gives a lovely glow – your legs will thank you for it! At the moment I'm loving Charlotte Tilbury Supermodel Body.

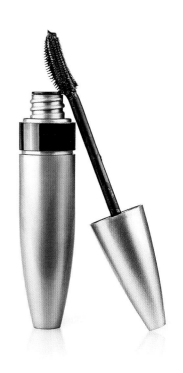

# Make-up Tips and Techniques

For me, flawless skin (or at least, as close as I can get) is the most important part of make-up. I prefer a dewy, glowing look, something very natural. But a matte look can be really striking as well. Whatever your preference, your skin should always look like your skin – not caked in make-up. I am prone to the odd break-out so I have become a master at making my skin look its best!

## Preparation

The key is continually looking after your skin and, of course, your daily skincare regime is an important part of this – when you're taking care of your skin and using the products and treatments most suited to your skin type, less and less work will go into making your skin look flawless! But if I have time before applying make-up, I would use a face mask or a light exfoliator before starting.

Then, apply a good-quality moisturiser – this doesn't necessarily mean expensive. Just make sure that it's suited to your skin type. Again, I use Image Skincare Prevention moisturiser – it's nice and light, and leaves my skin with a matte finish, acting as a good primer for my make-up so sometimes I don't need to use a primer. It also contains SPF (factor 32), which is vital. If your moisturiser doesn't have a high enough SPF, you may need to apply an SPF product separately to make sure your skin is getting the protection it needs.

If needed, I apply an illuminating primer all over my face – Charlotte Tilbury's Wonderglow is my favourite at the moment. If you prefer a matte finish, you should try the Urban Decay primers. Then you're ready to get started.

## Base

In my opinion, the most important element of a strong make-up look is a flawless base. It's so important to get this right, otherwise it throws everything else off. For example, if the colour of your foundation doesn't match your skin tone exactly, then that's all you'll see no matter how gorgeous you make your eyes or lips look. I think it's the hardest thing

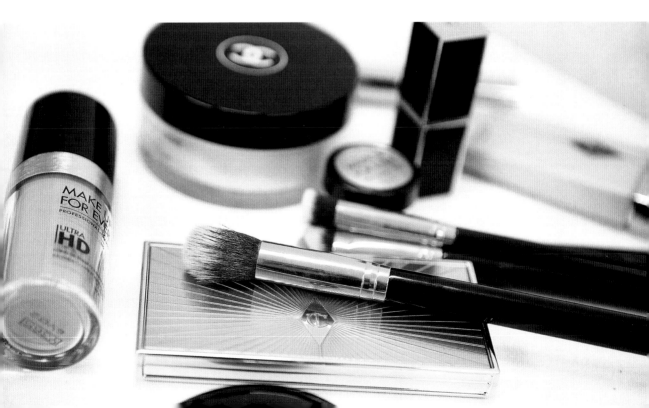

to perfect, but with a few well-chosen products you'll be on your way to gorgeous skin. There are four main things to consider when it comes to base: foundation, concealer, powder and contouring.

## Foundation

Always test your foundation on the side of your neck and coming up onto your face, rather than on the back of your hand – this way you can see if it's the same colour for both. The reason I apply some colour to my neck as well as my face is to make sure that it matches the colour of my body if I'm wearing tan and doesn't look too dark in comparison.

I use a fibre-optic foundation brush – you can use your fingers if you prefer, but I find that foundation stays in place longer when I use a brush. Apply small amounts at a time and buff into the skin in small circular motions.

## Concealer

You should have two types of concealer in your make-up bag: a light-reflecting one for around your eye area and a more opaque one for spots/blemishes. I find that a yellow-based concealer works best for me when it comes to covering blemishes and redness around my nose – I love The Retoucher by Charlotte Tilbury. For my eyes, I use one that's a few shades lighter than my skin tone.

## Powder

I then apply a powder to set the base. I use a nude pressed powder, but you can use a loose powder if you prefer.

## Contouring

Contouring is one of my favourite elements of a make-up look, as it can really accentuate your features. I think people can go a little overboard sometimes; soft and subtle is much better.

I use a bronzer and a small powder brush – you can use a cream concealer or foundation, but for everyday wear, powder is perfect. Also, creamy products can be time-consuming to apply and can end up looking heavy and artificial. Remember, the most important thing is to look like the best version of yourself – not to look completely different.

My favourite product for contouring is Charlotte Tilbury Filmstar Bronze & Glow. This compact also contains a powder highlighter that I use after I finish my whole face – if I do it before then, bits of eye make-up can fall down on my cheeks, making them look dirty, so it's best to wait until the very end.

Blush is the final stage of contouring. All you have to do is smile and apply your blusher to the apples of your cheeks. As with the bronzer above, use a small amount first and add as you go. I like to use a natural-looking, peachy blusher during the day and a brighter pink shade for evening. My go-to picks are anything by theBalm – they have so many beautiful colours. I like the Nars ones too.

## HOW TO CONTOUR

* Think of where the sun would naturally hit your face. Apply the product around your hairline and down either side of your nose.

* For definition on your cheekbones, apply it right underneath them. Use the line across from the top of your ear to your lip as a guideline, but never going down as far as your lip.

* You can also apply it underneath your jawline.

* Always start off lighter and apply more as needed – it's easier to add some than take some away.

# Brows

I always fill in my brows before I start on my eye make-up. I use an eyeshadow and angled brush rather than a pencil, as I prefer the finish that this gives, but it's totally up to you what you use. Just make sure you get a perfect match for your colouring. Brows frame your face, so it's important to get them right – make sure to refer back to Nilam's tips on page 171 for achieving the right shape, and, when it comes to make-up, she has more advice to offer.

## Nilam's top tips for styling your brows

You wouldn't leave the house without styling your hair in some way and the same should go for your brows – they need care and attention to look great too. Even those who are blessed with dense hair and perfectly shaped brows should, at the very least, brush them into place. The finish of the brow is key! Clients are often surprised that I layer many different make-up products and techniques to make their brows look textured and natural.

✧　　Don't over-colour-in brows. Block brows or brows that look too solid look unnatural. Remember, texture is the key to looking natural. You should still be able to see the hairs on a glamorous dark brow. Stand away from the mirror to ensure you can still see texture.

✧　　Do enhance your natural shape by adding make-up to lengthen or lift your brow, for example. We are not all lucky enough to have hair where we need it, so you can cheat your way to the perfect shape.

✧　　Use an angled brush with powders or creams or a superfine pencil to mimic hair strokes. Make sure your lines aren't too hard. Keep your colour within the hairs and only fill in the gaps. You can use a variety of products and still get a natural look – layering small amounts will help you achieve this. Practice makes perfect.

☆ Don't have an extreme shape, colour or size. If your brows are too arched, too dark, too big or too skinny, they will look OTT! I would allow one extreme. For example, you can have a fairly big brow but you can't have it big *and* dark. The most common mistakes are:

- Using the wrong colour powder or pencil: this is a big mistake but an easy one to fix. Make sure you use the colour that is most similar to your hair tone and you won't go wrong.

- Using too much make-up: your brows should not enter the room before you.

Although I like to see the effort people put into their brows, your brows should take no more than two minutes to style each day. Only fill in the areas that are missing.

## Eyeliner

Eyeliner can be a tricky thing to get right but practice makes perfect. It's definitely a key part of my everyday make-up look – I always use liner on my top lash line because it really opens up my eyes and makes them look bigger. Then I opt for a heavier lined eye, lining the bottom lashline and maybe even a winged look, for a bit more drama on a night out.

There are so many different types of liners available – pencil, liquid, gel – and I like to switch it up between them to achieve different looks. I love the liquid ones with the brush applicator, like the Rimmel Glam Eyes Liquid Liner, as they are easy to use, but I also use a fluid liner with a separate brush – although this is definitely more difficult to apply. You can also use an eyeshadow, which creates a much softer lined look.

## HOW TO APPLY EYELINER

* Use a very fine liner brush or an angled brush – again, I like the Callanberry range.

* Apply along the top lash line making sure to keep to the shape of your eye – the best thing to do is to use your own lash line as a guide. Start with a thin line which you can build on, depending on how dramatic you want your look to be. It's then time to do the flick – look in the mirror and choose where you want the flick to be.

* Make a little mark and bring the liner in to connect to the line you drew above the lash line.

* Match it on the other side – this can be difficult but, with practice, it gets easier.

* Always use a dry cotton bud to fix any little mistakes that you make.

## Red lips

Red lips look amazing, but as it's a very high-maintenance look, it isn't one to use if you need something to last a full day.

If my outfit is a little bit plain, I wear a red lip with it because I think this can dress it up! I always use a red lipstick with a blue tone because orange tones don't really suit me – it's important that you pick the right shade for you. It's a bit trial-and-error at first, so you need to go into a make-up counter and try lots of different shades until you find the perfect one. One of my favourites is MAC Ruby Woo.

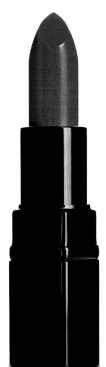

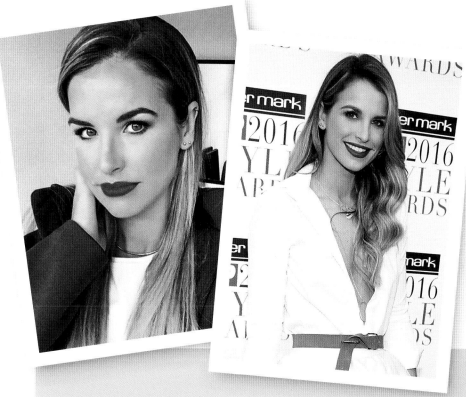

*If my outfit is a little bit plain, I wear a red lip with it because I think this can dress it up!*

## HOW TO DO A RED LIP

* For base/eyes/cheeks, I like to go with a natural look – see Look One on page 189.

* Use a red lip liner to line your lips – I sometimes draw a line slightly outside my natural lip line to make my lips look a little bit bigger. This takes a bit of practice but can be really effective if you want a fuller pout. You do have to be careful not to cheat too much by exaggerating your natural lip line, as this can end up looking really unnatural – remember, we want to enhance what you already have, not make you look like someone else (especially if that someone is a clown!).

* Then, fill in your lips with the liner because it will act as a really good colour base and will make your lipstick last longer.

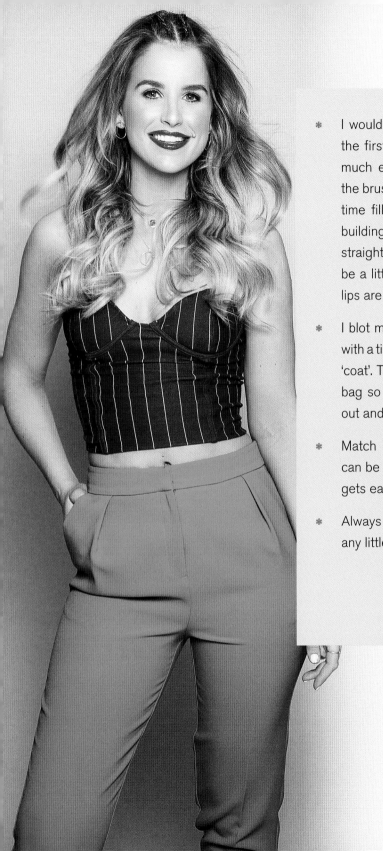

* I would always use a lip brush for the first application of lipstick. It's much easier, as the small size of the brush means you can take your time filling in your lips slowly and building up the colour. And applying straight from the lipstick bullet can be a little messy, especially if your lips are on the thin side.

* I blot my first application of colour with a tissue and then apply another 'coat'. Then, I pop my lipstick in my bag so I can touch it up when I'm out and about.

* Match it on the other side – this can be difficult but, with practice, it gets easier.

* Always use a dry cotton bud to fix any little mistakes that you make.

# Look One: Daytime Smoky

I don't always have time to do a full make-up look, especially if I'm rushing out to meetings during the week. I end up wearing a lot of make-up because of my job so sometimes I just really want to keep it natural. I depend on this look a lot, which only takes ten minutes and is so easy to do.

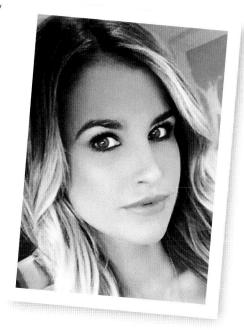

## Base

I apply a light foundation with my fibre-optic brush and apply concealer to where it's needed, usually under my eyes. Then I apply a powder to set my foundation, followed by a bit of bronzer and highlighter on my cheekbones and nose. Then I finish my base with some blusher on the apples of my cheeks.

## Eyes

When it comes to eyeshadow for this look, I opt for a taupey-brown shade, nothing too dark, which gives me nice definition. Using a dome-shaped brush, start on the outer corner of your lid making sure to tap off any excess shadow beforehand, and blend into the socket. Repeat this step, building up the colour slowly, until you're happy with it. Then apply a slightly darker shadow underneath the lower lash line using an angled brush and blend to achieve a smoky effect.

On the waterline and on the top lash line, I use a gel liner and a fine liner brush. Make sure you don't have too much liner on the brush and remember to take your time. I often wing the liner – I pick the exact point on either side where the wing will start and make a small mark with my brush there, and then fill in the line slowly towards my lash line. This way you know that both lines will be even when you're finished.

## Lashes

I curl my top and bottom lashes and apply a generous amount of mascara. To avoid clumping, I use a lash/brow comb and brush through my lashes after each application – I like to use two coats.

## Lips

I like to go with a natural lip for this look so I pick a matte lipstick in a soft pink shade, and apply a layer of gloss in a matching shade on top because I like a glossier lip. Quick mirror check, and I'm good to go!

### Product list

**Foundation:** Make Up For Ever Ultra HD Foundation

**Concealer:** Make Up For Ever Lift Concealer

**Powder:** db Face Cosmetics – Nude Pressed Powder

**Bronzer:** db Face Cosmetics – Congo

**Blusher:** Inglot Freedom System

**Highlighter:** theBalm – Mary-Lou Manizer

**Brows:** db Face Cosmetics – Eyeshadow 225

**Eyeshadow:** Urban Decay Naked 1 palette – Naked (crease), Buck (lash line)

**Liner:** MAC Pro Longwear Fluidline – Blacktrack

**Mascara:** Bobbi Brown Smokey Eye – Black

**Lipstick:** MAC – Blankety

**Lip gloss:** Daniel Sandler Super Gloss – Super Nectar

# Look Two: Glam Daytime

This is the look I go for when I want to make a bit of an effort, but still achieve a fairly soft look – it's perfect for attending weddings or going to the races. And it photographs really well. (This is the look I'm wearing on the book cover!)

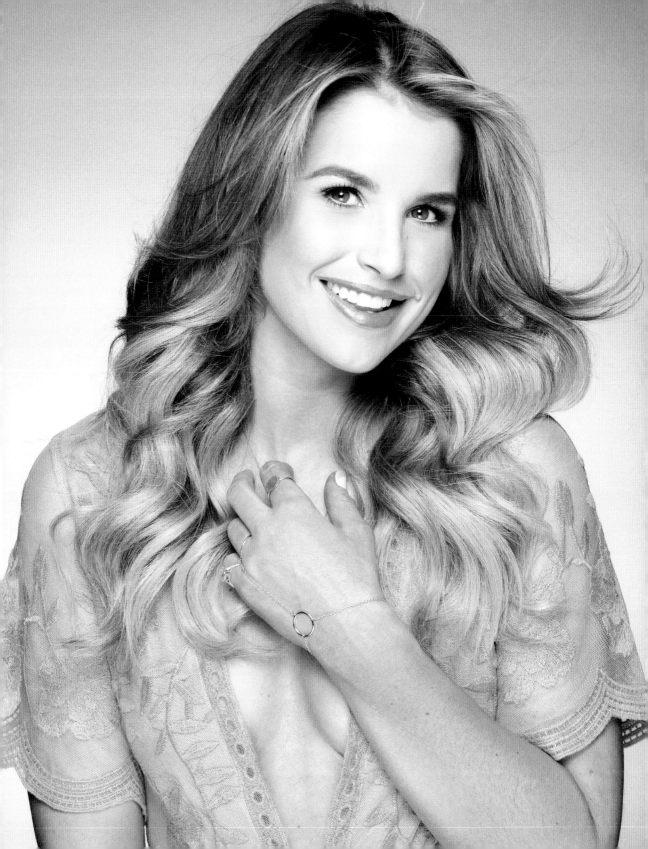

## Base

The first thing I apply to my face is moisturiser – for this look, I like to choose one that has a little bit of shimmer to it to give my skin a healthy glow. MAC Strobe Cream is perfect for this.

Next is my foundation – I apply this with a stippling brush to achieve an airbrushed effect, making sure that it's really well blended. Next I add a bit of concealer under my eyes and on any areas of redness on my face – I like to use a really light concealer for this. Then I use a cream concealer if there are any blemishes I need to cover up.

To set my make-up, I apply a bit of loose powder all over my face using a big brush – and then, using a smaller brush, apply a layer of powder under my eyes to set the concealer there.

Next up: contouring! I apply contour powder on my temples, under my cheekbones, and on my jawline and neckline, making sure to blend it thoroughly (so I don't end up with stripes across my face!). The Charlotte Tilbury Bronze & Glow palette is a product I love because it includes a highlighter as well as a contour shade. If I have this palette in my bag, I'll add the highlighter shade on the top of my cheekbones, on my brow bones and sometimes on my nose and cupid's bow.

And for the finishing touch to my base I add a pop of peachy-pink blusher – this is the perfect shade for Irish skin tones as it looks so natural.

## Eyes

I fill in my brows with pencil and then brush them through with a gel, such as Gimme Brow from the Benefit range. Another make-up artist tip: spray a bit of hairspray on a clean mascara wand and then brush this through your eyebrows to set them and keep them tidy. As for eyeshadow, I keep it fairly natural – applying a light cream shade as a base on my eyelids and then a taupe or brown shade in the crease and on the lower lash line. For an extra bit of sparkle, I dab on a little bit of shimmery eyeshadow on the inner corners of my eyes. Then I apply black gel liner with an angled brush – this look is a little more daytime so I would just apply a thin line on my top lash line, but for a night-time look I would wing it out. And to finish off my eyes, I'll add two coats of black mascara to my top and bottom lashes. False eyelashes can make your eyes really pop – for this look, I like to wear some individual lashes scattered on my top lash line.

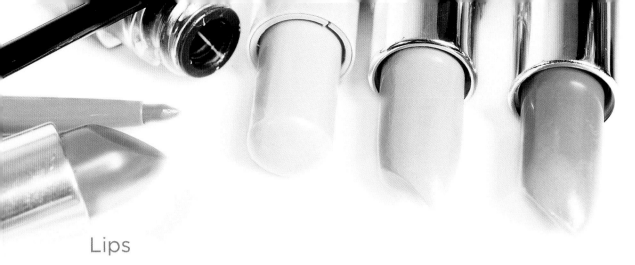

## Lips

Again, I like to keep my lip colour fairly natural for this look. Pillow Talk from the Charlotte Tilbury range is one of my favourite products at the moment – it's a lip liner in a really soft, delicate pink and I absolutely love it. I line my lips with this colour and then fill in my lips with the liner too – a great base for my lipstick, and it also means there's a bit of colour there when the lipstick starts to wear off. Then I apply a pinky-nude lipstick and slap on some lip gloss for the finishing touch.

### Product list

**Moisturiser:** MAC Strobe Cream

**Foundation:** Make Up For Ever HD Ultra 365.

**Concealer:** Charlotte Tilbury Retoucher (under eyes); MAC Studio Finish (imperfections)

**Powder:** Laura Mercier Loose Powder

**Contouring:** Charlotte Tilbury Bronze & Glow palette

**Blusher:** Charlotte Tilbury Cheek to Chic – Ecstasy

**Eyebrows:** MAC brow pencil – Lingering; Benefit Gimme Brow.

**Eye Shadow:** MAC Eye Shadow – Vanilla and Nylon; Urban Decay – Tease (Naked 2 palette)

**Eyeliner:** MAC Fluidline Eyeliner Gel – Blacktrack

**Mascara:** Urban Decay Perversion

**Lip liner:** Charlotte Tilbury Lip Cheat – Pillow Talk

**Lipstick:** Tom Ford – Blush Nude

**Lip gloss:** Charlotte Tilbury Lip Lustre – Seduction

# Look Three: Flawless Night-time

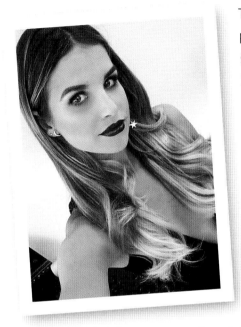

This is one of my all-time favourite make-up looks, perfect for parties and evenings out. And if you're going relatively simple with your outfit – maybe with your tried-and-trusted LBD – this look packs a lot of punch. And, you'll be glad to hear, it is relatively easy for anybody to recreate when you have the right blending brushes. It's a soft, well-blended smoky eye with a burgundy lip and will look beautiful on most skin tones. The burgundy lip is seen at fashion week almost every year for autumn–winter collections, so it's a pretty safe make-up look to keep you on-trend. Celebrities from Rihanna and J-Lo to Rosie Huntington-Whiteley and Scarlett Johansson have worn this kind of look on the red carpet over and over again, and it always looks amazing.

If a dark lip scares you, though, just substitute the lip colour for something in a nude pink tone (I suggest MAC Blankety), which also complements this look perfectly.

## Base

To ensure my skin is looking extra-flawless, I apply a face balm before applying my foundation using a stipple brush. I put concealer under my eyes and sweep it across the cheekbones to use it as a highlighter. Then I set the foundation with some translucent powder.

Next step is a bronzing powder to add contouring, and I use a plum-coloured blusher to complement my lipstick shade. Finally, I highlight the higher planes of the face – the cheekbones, cupid's bow, jawline and slightly above and below the brows.

# Eyes

I apply eyeshadow in a charcoal brown shade through my eyebrows with a liner brush and then use a gel to set them.

On my eyelids, I use a base to keep the shadow in place, which you can apply using your finger to ensure it covers the lid all the way from the lash line to the brow. Then I use a white kohl pencil on the waterline to brighten up my eyes. Next, I apply a base-colour eyeshadow – I usually use a taupe or light brown over my lid – before sweeping the transition colour, a smoky brown, on the socket line and wrapping it all the way around the eye with a big fluffy blending brush.

Then I deepen the crease using a darker eyeshadow, which I also apply on the lower lash line using a slanted liner brush. I finish the eyes with a gel liner on my top lashline with a flick and lots of mascara.

# Lips

For the perfect burgundy lip, I start by applying a primer to keep everything in place. After this, I carefully line and then fill in my lips using a lip pencil in a matching shade and, finally, a matte lipstick.

## Product list

**Primer:** Clarins Beauty Flash Balm

**Foundation:** Make Up For Ever HD Foundation

**Concealer:** MAC Pro Longwear Concealer

**Powder:** MAC Mineralize Skinfinish

**Bronzer:** Bobbi Brown Bronzing Powder, in medium

**Blusher:** MAC Powder Blush – Plum Foolery

**Highlighter:** MAC Mineralize Skinfinish – Soft and Gentle

**Eyeshadow:** Mac Pro Longwear Paint Pot – Painterly (base); Mac Eye Shadow – Blanc Type (base-colour), Sketch (crease/lower lash line); Urban Decay Naked 1 – Buck (transition)

**Brows:** MAC Charcoal Brown eye shadow; Benefit Gimme Brows

**Eyeliner:** Inglot AMC Eyeliner Gel – 77
**Mascara:** Revlon Ultra Volume Mascara – Black
**Lips:** MAC Prep + Prime Lip; MAC Lip pencil – Burgundy; MAC Lipstick – Diva

# Look Four: Casual Daytime

On my days off, I often go make-up free. But if I am out and about – maybe lunch with friends or an afternoon at the shops – I like to go with a soft, low-key look. These free days are usually when I pay my skin extra-special attention, so I might apply a clay mask or exfoliate and make my skin look extra bright before I open my make-up bag.

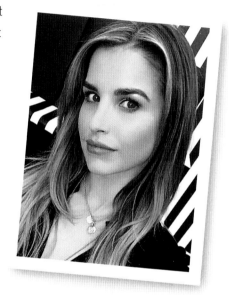

## Base

After I've applied my moisturiser, I like to use a bit of primer, as I think this makes my skin look as smooth and radiant as possible. Next, it's foundation – I use a lightweight formula on days like these, as glossy, natural skin is the look I'm going for – and bit of concealer where it's needed (usually under my eyes if it's been a busy week!). Then I dab some bronzer on the parts of my face where the sun would naturally hit me – my cheekbones, my temples and a little on my nose. A bit of peachy blusher goes on my cheeks next – I like to use a cream blusher for this look. And to complete my base, I apply some powder to set my make-up but only to my T-zone so as not to dull the nice glowing finish I've created.

## Eyes

I use a cream eyeshadow in a light gold colour on my lids, and then I add a darker bronze tone on the crease. Again, I'm keeping it simple so I tend to be drawn towards products that I can apply with my fingers. Next, I use a pen liner to apply a soft flick to my top lashline, and then I add two coats of black mascara.

## Lips

I line my lips using a light pink liner and then pucker up with a moisturising lipstick in a summery pink shade – I definitely don't want anything high-maintenance on a day off!

### Product list

**Primer:** Benefit Porefessional
**Foundation:** Charlotte Tilbury Wonderglow
**Concealer:** MAC Pro Longwear Concealer in NW20
**Bronzer:** Charlotte Tilbury Beach Stick – Ibiza
**Blusher:** Bobbi Brown Pot Rouge for Lips & Cheeks – Fresh Melon
**Powder:** MAC Mineralize Skinfinish, in medium plus
**Eyeshadow:** Bobbi Brown Longwear Cream Shadow – Sandy Gold (lids), Beach Bronze (crease)
**Liner:** Make Up For Ever Graphic Liner
**Mascara:** Benefit They're Real! Lengthening Mascara
**Lip Liner:** Charlotte Tilbury – Pillow Talk
**Lipstick:** Charlotte Tilbury K.I.S.S.I.N.G. – Valentine

# Look Five:
# Night-Time Smoky Eye

A smoky eye gives a simple outfit like a white T-shirt and jeans the wow factor, and it looks absolutely gorgeous when you're dolled up to the nines too. I tend to go with quite a matte finish on my skin for this look – but I do my eyes first, just in case bits of eye make-up end up on my cheeks.

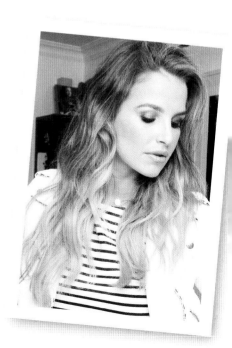

## Eyes

I start off by applying a matte base on my eyelid – you can use a primer for this or even a cream eyeshadow in a pale colour.

When it comes to a smoky eye, dark greys and browns are most common but I love to see people change it up with navy, purple or dark green. I like to pick the colour I'm going with and then choose two or three shades to blend together to achieve a really rich colour. One of my favourites is a coppery-green smoky eye – I blend a beautiful sparkly emerald-green shadow and an eyeshadow in a bronze shade.

Once my base shade is in place, I start by applying the green shadow with a dome-shaped brush – a fairly thin layer to my eyelid, more generously to the socket line and blending out to the outer corners of my eyes. I build up the colour slowly, making sure to buff with the brush. Then I use the bronze shade in the same way, blending with the brush or fingers. And I just keep building and blending with each colour – checking my look carefully in the mirror as I go – until I'm happy with the effect.

I also use a smaller brush to add a smudge of shadow under my eye, again making sure to blend really well. And then I use pencil eyeliner in a chocolate-brown shade on my lower waterline to add to the soft, smoky look.

Remember, it's supposed to look a bit messy – that's part of the appeal of this look – so don't worry about it looking perfect. Smudgy and sultry is what we're going for!

I complete my eye make-up with a flick of black gel liner and lots of volumising black mascara. Then I do a careful tidy-up around my eyes, wiping away any stray bits of eyeshadow that might be on my cheeks, before I get started on my base.

## Base

I use a brush to apply foundation to make sure the finish is polished and concealer under my eyes and on any blemishes. Then I set with loose powder.

I keep my brows fairly natural so will just fill them in with pencil. The eyes are the focus with this look, so I'll only add a small amount of blusher on my cheeks, to make sure I'm not looking too pale, and some highlighter on my cheekbones.

## Lips

I like to keep the focus on my eyes for this look, so will finish off with a nude lip.

### Product suggestions

**Foundation:** Make Up For Ever HD Foundation

**Concealer:** Charlotte Tilbury Retoucher

**Powder:** Laura Mercier Translucent Loose Setting Powder

**Highlighter:** theBalm – Mary-Lou Manizer

**Blusher:** Benefit CORALista

**Eyeshadow:** Charlotte Tilbury Luxury Palette – The Rebel (pop shade); Charlotte Tilbury Colour Chameleon – Golden Quartz

**Liner:** MAC Eye Kohl – Costa Riche

**Brows:** MAC brow pencil – Lingering

**Mascara:** Revlon Ultra Volume – Black

**Lip Liner:** Charlotte Tilbury – Pillow Talk

**Lipstick:** Charlotte Tilbury K.I.S.S.I.N.G. – Nude Kate

# Hair

I am obsessed with good hair. I think if you're having a good hair day, you're on to a winner. However, I can be super lazy when it comes to taking care of and styling my hair. I get it done so often for work that when it comes to styling it myself I tend to go for a natural look. But if you take care of your hair, and it's cut and styled in a look that works for you, you can have good hair without too much hard work (meaning you can have an extra few minutes in bed instead of having to battle with your locks in the morning!). I also swear by a silk pillowcase, it tames the overnight frizz!

My hair is naturally wavy and prone to frizziness. I love wearing it long because it's so much easier to manage – and the length means I can style it lots of different ways. When I was a teenager, I went for that very bleached-out look, which was not a good idea.

First, the colour did not suit me at all – it totally washed out my skin – and, second, it totally ruined my hair. Bleached hair needs a lot of TLC, and I didn't make the effort to do this (lazy, remember!). I still like to keep my hair blonde but now I like it to look as natural as possible. I never get a full head of highlights anymore. I was delighted when the balayage trend started – dark roots, lighter ends – because it meant I didn't need to get my roots done as often, giving my hair a break, and I actually prefer the look, even now. I only have my hair coloured every six months at the moment, and I opt for scattered highlights with a few at the front.

When I do my own hair, I either straighten it and put it into a sleek high pony or curl it and leave it down. I like messy curls the best, which is handy because I'm not a pro when it comes to using curling tongs so I always end up with a beachy vibe anyway.

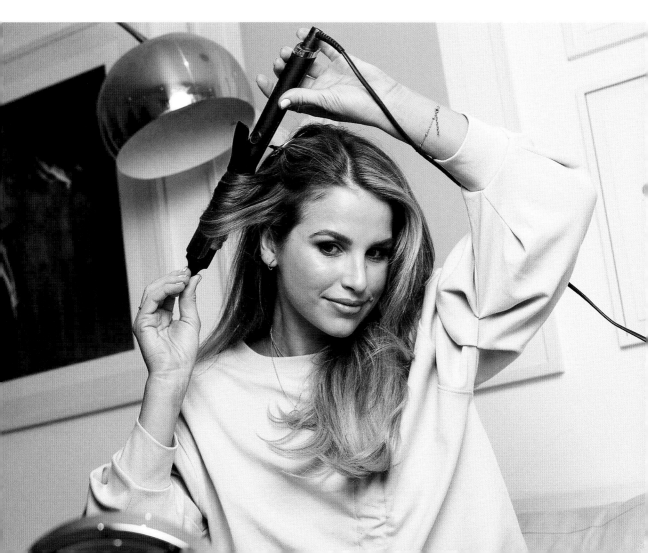

One of the big things when it comes to feeling happy with your hair is finding the right hair stylist. What you need is someone who listens to you and asks the right questions – there's no point in moving forward with a high-maintenance hairstyle if you don't have time to style it or (if you're anything like me) you don't enjoy spending too much time on your hair. I think personal recommendations are great – don't be afraid to quiz people whose hairstyles you admire about what salon they go to! Make sure you have a good long chat with the stylist during your first visit or when you want to make a big change, and don't be afraid to tell them, or just try someone or somewhere else, if you're not happy with what they're doing for your hair. It also goes without saying that you should never make a dramatic change to your hair when you're going through any kind of personal drama – getting a funky new look after a break-up can be fun, but I've had a few friends who regretted an impulsive hair decision!

## My hair kit

### Shampoo and conditioner

I swear by a good shampoo and conditioner – my hair is quite dry and needs extra love because I colour it, so I make sure that the products I use suit my hair type. There are a lot of different brands and types to choose from, so it can take a lot of trial and error to find the right ones. I always think it's a good idea to ask advice from your hairdresser, who should be able to give you guidance on what your hair needs and what products will do the trick. My favourite brands are Kevin Murphy, Redken and Kerastase, which I buy from my hair salon. They're a little more expensive, but I think it's worth investing in the right products, especially the ones that do the job of cleaning and nourishing your hair.

### Oil

I always use an oil on my hair after I wash it – at the moment, I'm using Moroccanoil Treatment. This makes it easier to brush and it looks much sleeker when it dries.

## Dry shampoo

Dry shampoo is a must for every girl. It's best not to wash your hair every day if you can help it, as it gets rid of the natural oils. And if you have long hair like mine, washing and drying it takes up a lot of time that you could spend doing something else. I wash mine three to four times a week and use dry shampoo on the days in between to stop it from looking greasy. A particular favourite of mine is Kevin Murphy Doo Over, but the Batiste range is brilliant as well (and very budget-friendly). However, make sure not to use dry shampoo too often – it is not a substitute for cleaning your hair, and if over-used it could affect your hair's natural balance.

## Sea salt spray

If I'm feeling lazy, or I want to give my hair a break, I don't bother with a blow-dry and let my hair dry naturally – this also gives my hair a much-needed break from constant heat and styling. I just load it up with some sea salt spray and scrunch it with my hands. I love the Kevin Murphy Hair Resort. Other great products are the Toni & Guy Sea Salt Texturising Spray and the Bumble and Bumble Surf Spray. Sea salt spray is one of my favourite products, as it gives my hair a really natural, textured beach wave look.

## Protein spray

I use protein spray to give my hair a little more strength, as it takes a battering with the constant washing and heat and colour treatments I get. A protein spray contains keratin, which strengthens the hair against breakage, and my favourite product is Redken Extreme CAT Protein Spray.

## Heat protectant

As I use so many heating appliances on my hair – hairdryers, straighteners, rollers and tongs – I make sure to use a heat protectant. The silicones in the protectants act a little like sun protection for our skin, protecting the cuticle of the hair. They are also really good for moisturising the hair, which again is important if you use a lot of heat styling.

## Hair masks

To really keep my hair in good condition, I use a hair mask once a week. I try not to use one that weighs down my hair or makes it feel greasy. I love Kerastase products, and their mask is brilliant, but also recommended is the Aussie 3 Minute Miracle Reconstructor – it's a bargain!

## Hairspray

Hairspray is an absolute necessity, especially if your hair is prone to frizzing. Nothing worse than slaving over a hairstyle or spending ages in the salon, and then having to sit in a corner because you're worried about it falling down. My faves are Kevin Murphy's Anti Gravity spray and L'Oréal's Elnett Satin.

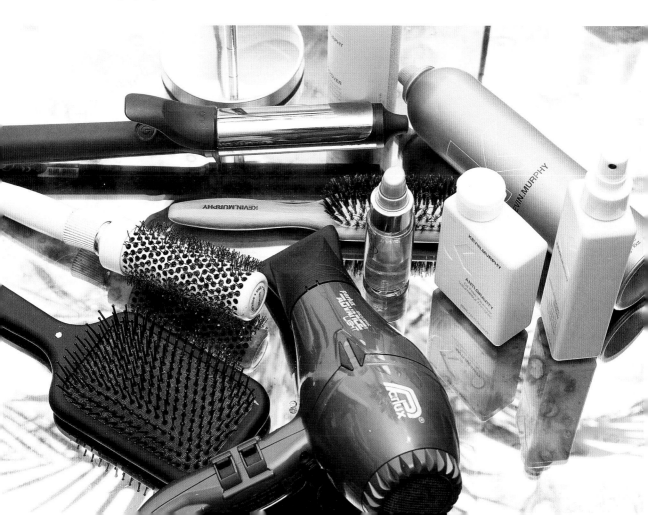

## Hair brushes

Brushing my hair has been a hatred of mine ever since I was a child – I had many an argument with my mother when she tried to brush my hair. I wore a hairband with my hair down until about the age of twelve and never had a ponytail because that would only prolong the painful experience of someone touching my hair!

I am very particular about what hairbrush I use because of this. I always have a few rounded barrel brushes that I use to blow-dry my hair with, as these dry it straighter. My everyday brush is one with soft bristles. I like it because it's gentle on my hair, especially when I'm wearing extensions (really important – more on this later). I also like the Wet Brush and the Tangle Teezer, as they eliminate the pain but still get rid of the knots in my hair.

## Styling tools

I think it's really important to have a good hairdryer. You use it a lot so it makes sense to invest. I swear by the Parlux range of hairdryers, which are brilliant. I have a collection of three of these now because I can't bear to be without one – one for travelling and one each in my houses in London and Dublin. One is still going strong after eight years, so it was well worth the investment.

I rarely wear my hair straight – if I do, it usually means I'm having a lazy day! When I do straighten my hair, I would use my heat protection products, blow-dry it first with a rounded brush and then use my GHD hair straightener. Although GHD products are expensive, they last for years and are the best straightening tool on the market.

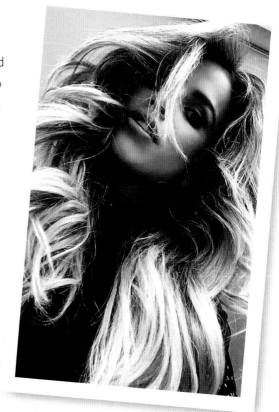

*I love wearing my hair long because it's so much easier to manage.*

Curly hair is my thing, though – whether it's a bouncy curl, beach-wave or messy look, it's my favourite hairstyle. I've used and bought so many curling tongs and my favourite is from the GHD range – it holds the curl better than any others I've tried. I also have a curling wand with a medium-sized barrel, which means the curl won't be too tight. The wand would be my tool of preference for everyday styling as it gives a better beachy wave than tongs.

Heated rollers are pretty old school, but they do give great volume. Just remember to buy medium to large rollers – otherwise you'll end up with very tight curls. When I'm getting ready to go on a night out, I'll blow-dry my hair and then pop in my heated rollers – I have the O Rollers from Cloud Nine – while I'm doing my make-up.

## Hair treatments

Because I have my hair coloured, I find it gets really dry, really quickly. When I'm at the salon, I always ask them to use a treatment when I'm having my hair washed – again, your hairdresser is the person who'll know best what your hair needs, and sometimes you even get treated to a lovely head massage. Some treatments are used to restore moisture to the hair, others – like silver shampoo – are used to maintain your hair colour. A new discovery that I love is a salon treatment called Olaplex that works on repairing your hair.

I do lots of treatments at home too, at least once a week. Usually you have to leave them in for at least fifteen minutes, so it can be a nice excuse to put your feet up – and maybe you'll decide to do your nails while you're waiting for it to take effect. My favourites are hot oil treatments, which make my hair feel really soft. I'm using products from the Redken, Kerastase and Kevin Murphy ranges at the moment, but there are lots available from pharmacies and supermarkets.

## Extensions

A question I'm asked a lot is what type of hair extensions I use. At this stage, I think I've probably tried them all!

When I was a teenager I used the dreaded clip-ins, which made me look like I had a mullet. But this didn't deter me. I wore them proudly regardless, with the clips clearly visible! Now, I sometimes use the Easilocks clip-in extensions – a much more modern version with very discreet clips – when I want more volume in my hair or longer length.

Clip-ins work well if you only want extensions for big nights out or events – but I adore having extensions all the time. I have become a little addicted and don't even leave a day between getting them taken out and new ones put in.

For the past seven years, I have used Great Lengths, which stylist Ceira Lambert puts in for me every five or six months. The hair quality is really good and they hold a curl or style well. I have quite long hair anyway so I just use the extensions to add volume.

Some people believe that extensions ruin your hair but I don't find this to be the case if you choose the right ones. I have had mishaps in the past and it's why I stick with Ceira as she has always looked after my extensions, ensuring to keep my hair looking great. I actually think the extensions protect my hair from the constant styling my work requires. But do not get extensions where glue is used to apply them – I made that mistake years ago, and not only was my hair incredibly matted, it was very sore and time-consuming to get them removed. Never again!

There are so many types of extensions available and you can get different ones for different types of hair. Great Lengths use a keratin bond, which works best in my hair. Easilocks use a removal bond that uses no heat, and a lot of people go for this type too.

## Hairstyles

I wanted to let you know how to do a few of my favourite hairstyles at home, though I have roped in a couple of my favourite hairdressers to help me out. My best friend and hairdresser Matthew Feeney used to do my hair all the time in Dublin, but I stole him from Ireland and he now lives with me in London, so he is my go-to person there. I will never have another bad hair day as long as he lives with me! In Dublin, my favourite person to go to is Carla Rose McQuillan from The Space in Drumcondra.

## A sleek pony

A sleek pony is so easy to do and suits everyone. It's a great daytime look, but it totally works for a night out too.

After I've washed and blow-dried my hair, I use a straightener to make sure it's poker straight. The hard part is fastening/securing the pony with no bumps – I like mine really high, too, which makes it even harder. I just throw my head forward and gather all of my hair in my hand. I then use a brush to smooth it out, but it has to be a soft-bristle brush for me.

When I have gathered the pony, I use a bobbin to tie up my hair and tighten it as much as I can. I then use a strand of hair from the ponytail to wrap around the bobbin, so you can't see it, and pin it in using bobby pins. Then I spray it with hairspray and make it more sleek, using my hands to smooth it back.

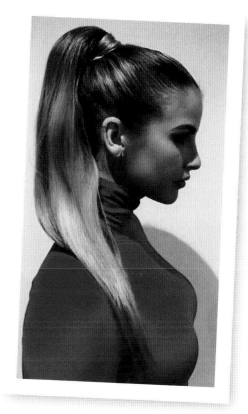

*A great daytime look but it works for night too.*

## Bouncy curls

This is my signature hairstyle – I find it hard to say anything other than 'bouncy blow-dry' when I'm at the hairdresser's. I think it's such a great look for any time of day, any occasion, and instantly makes you look done up even if you have no make-up on. Matthew Feeney is the king of bouncy blow-dries, so this is how he creates the look for me.

First of all, he preps my hair with Kevin Murphy Anti Gravity while it's damp – he applies this to my roots to create volume. Next, he'll add some Wella Luxe Oil Reconstructive Elixir to my ends and extensions – this makes my hair really soft and keeps it from getting tangled. (It can also be used as a leave-in treatment.) And then he takes a dollop of Kevin

Murphy Hair Resort, rubs this on his hands and applies throughout my hair. This preps it for curling and creates a beachy, messy texture.

Then he blow-dries my hair using a rounded brush. And after that he'll work on it with the GHD Curve Wave Wand to achieve soft, natural-looking curls.

## Beach waves

I always have a beach-wave kind of look the day after a bouncy blow-dry. I just throw a load of product in it, sea salt spray and hairspray, and scrunch it all up in my hands.

If I haven't had a bouncy blow-dry the day before, I start from scratch. I wash and blow-dry my hair. Then I use the GHD conical wand to style my hair – but I make sure to leave the last two to three inches of my hair straight, so I don't get that bounce on the ends. And I'll either finish up with Hair Resort, which gives my hair a wetter, grittier texture, or Doo Over, which gives a fluffier look.

## Plaits

Plaits are back in style in a big way. I tend to get them done at the hairdresser's, as they can be quite fiddly, but there are two that I've mastered at home.

I'm a big fan of the messy side plait. Start by washing and blow-drying your hair – or you can do styles like this on day two as well. The messier your hair the better for this one. Pull

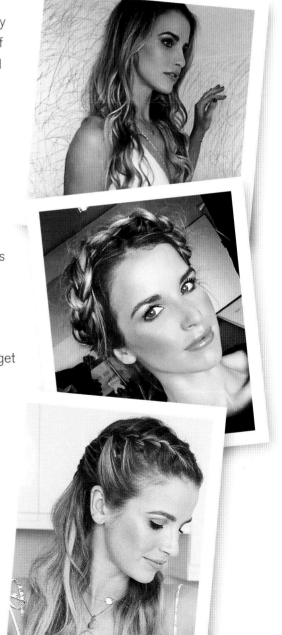

*Plaits are back in style in a big way.*

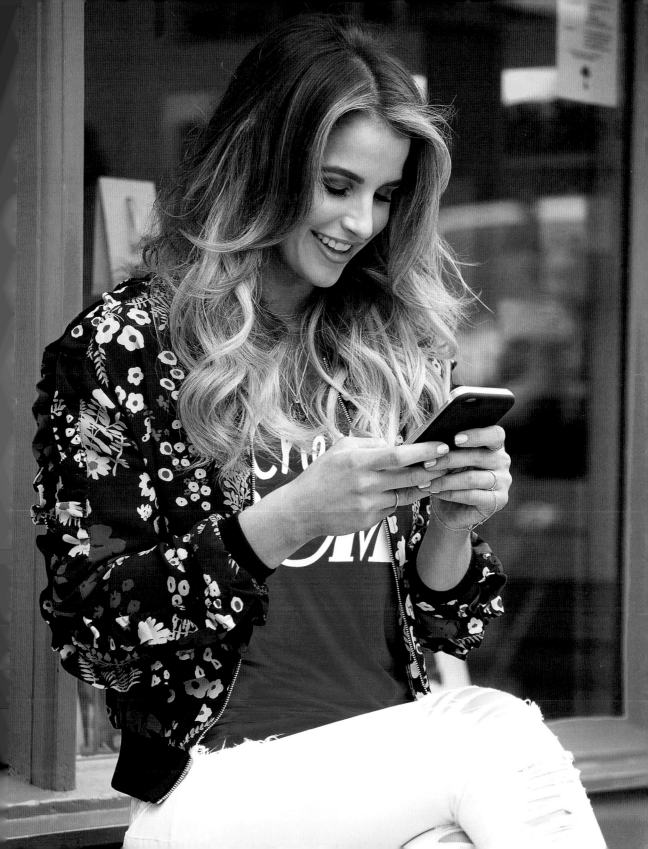

all of your hair over to one side to create a side parting and start the plait from the base of your neck, making sure it's quite loose. When you have finished your plait, pull at your hair to loosen the plait further. I like to leave bits of hair down at the front to frame my face and make it look a little undone.

## Messy bun

I usually do a messy bun a couple of days after I have washed my hair, when I'm too lazy to do anything else with it! For a neater style, it's best to do it with freshly washed and dried hair. Then use a tong to give your hair a slight wave. After that, pull your hair up into a ponytail using your fingers – this doesn't have to be completely smooth. Then get another bobbin, grab the pony and put it into a messy bun with little bits coming down – don't twist the pony: just throw it up.

## Messy up-do

All of my hairstyles start the same sort of way – it just goes to show that you don't need to be amazing at doing your hair: you just need to master a few basics.

If necessary, I wash and dry my hair and then curl it with my tongs. This one is actually better if you do it with unwashed hair but it will still work with washed hair. When it's curled, I back comb the top back part of my hair to give it volume. I then grab it into a low pony and tie it up, remembering to keep plenty of pieces down at the front of my hairline. You need lots of bobby pins for the next part. I do a sort of bun, but really messy, and instead of using a bobbin, I fasten it

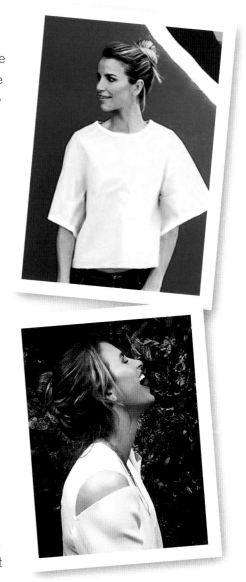

*This one is actually better if you do it with unwashed hair.*

with bobby pins instead. I then recurl the front parts of my hair that were left out and spray it all with hairspray.

## Sleek up-do

To me, Kim Kardashian is the queen of the sleek up-do – she never has a hair out of place. The good news is this style isn't difficult or time-consuming.

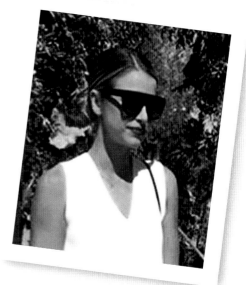

After drying my hair, I straighten it so that it's poker straight. I then use a comb with a metal point at the end to get a perfectly symmetrical side parting à la Kim. I get it into a low pony using a brush so there are no bumps in it, and then tie it really tightly. I then twirl the pony around to make it into a neat bun and use another bobbin to secure it. The key with this is loads of hairspray – it will make it extra sleek and keep it in place.

*This style isn't difficult or time-consuming.*

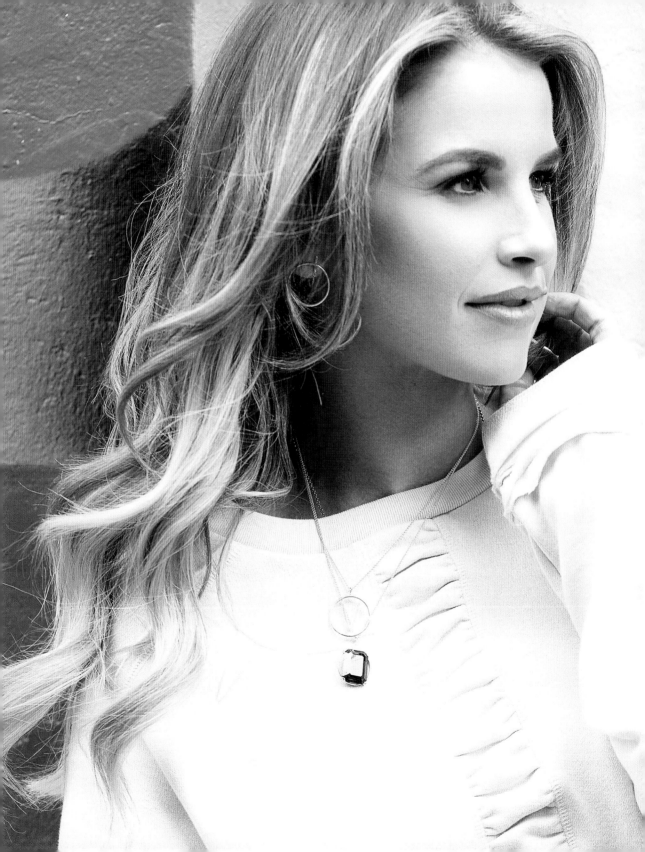

# Style

Style is different for everyone. While fashions might change, we all have different things we like and I love the individuality of it all. My style changes depending on what mood I'm in, but usually I sport a kind of androgynous look because I'm really a tomboy at heart. When I go out to events, I tend to dress up quite girly, and I love that look too. Instagram is a great way to keep up with fashion and get great tips. I often get ideas from the people I follow, and it's a brilliant way for me to discover new designers too. But the really important thing about style, regardless of what's in fashion at any moment, is to make sure that your clothes fit properly, that you are comfortable in them and that you wear them with confidence.

# Underwear

In order for your clothes to look good on your body, what's underneath has to be doing its job! Matching sets are great – and look fantastic when you have your clothes off – but I envy the girls who wear matching underwear every day, because I rarely do. It's more important that my underwear is giving me the support I need.

I have a million bras but always stick to my favourite ones. You can't underestimate the importance of wearing a bra that fits. My bra size has changed a few times over the years, and it turns out I was wearing the wrong size for a really long time, so now I make sure to get measured every year.

I have lots of different types of bras, but my favourite is an underwire style with a little bit of padding. Lace bras are totally

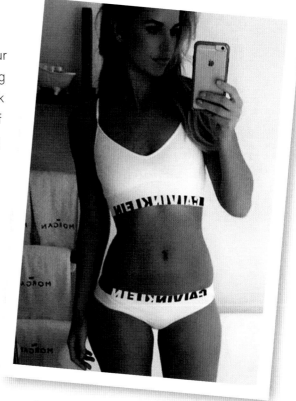

*Matching sets are great – and look fantastic when you have your clothes off.*

back in and they look great if you wear a low-cut top and your bra can be slightly seen. Nude underwear is not very sexy, but it's definitely a wardrobe staple for me, particularly because of my love of white clothes.

To me, there is nothing worse than seeing a knicker line through tight clothing. If I am wearing a very fitted dress or pair of trousers, I always wear a seamless thong. But for everyday wear, I like to opt for something more comfortable, usually cotton.

Spanx are also a must in my wardrobe. People think Spanx are just for making you look slimmer, but I wear them to create a smoother line if I'm wearing a floor-length gown.

I like a cute bodysuit, too, and have a few of those that I sometimes wear as tops with a blazer over it.

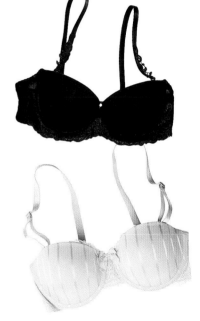

## UNDERWEAR STAPLES

* Bras (nude, black, white)

* Strapless bras (nude, black)

* Lace bras (white, black)

* Seamless thongs (nude, black, white)

* Spanx (nude, black)

# My Wardrobe Essentials

I am guilty of only wearing a small portion of the clothes in my wardrobe – on my days off, I always seem to grab the same things. When it comes to everyday wear, I tend to keep things fairly simple – skinny jeans or leather trousers with a crisp-white, baggy T-shirt, runners and a nice coat. Throw on a pair of heels instead of the runners and I'm dressed up for an evening out. But here are some of my basic must-have pieces.

## T-shirts

I always have black, white and light-grey short-sleeve cotton T-shirts. They go with everything and are so handy for any look.

## Jeans

I only ever wear skinny jeans – as they are most flattering for my shape – and I have about fifty pairs in all different colours, but, of course, I just wear my favourite ones all the time. My go-to blue pair cost me €20 in Zara, and I never take them off – I only wish I had bought a few more pairs of them. It can be difficult to find jeans to fit just right – I would recommend visiting a shop with lots of different brands and styles and asking for advice from the retail assistant. Bringing a very honest friend also helps! Don't be put off if the style you like is too long – it's much more

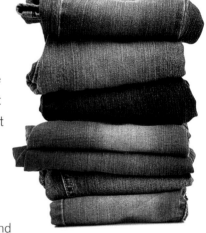

important for them to fit well around the waist and bum, and alterations to the length can be made easily at fairly low cost. I like to buy jeans that are pretty tight-fitting, as the last thing I want is for a new pair to be baggy around the bum and knees when the denim starts to stretch.

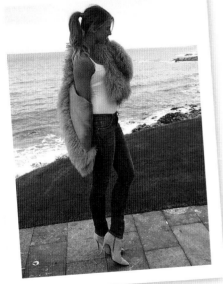

## Stripes for life

I am obsessed with any type of stripe, but I'm particularly partial to a navy and white combo. I have a lot of tops and jumpers in this nautical design and like wearing them with a khaki or army coat – I think

*I only ever wear skinny jeans as they are the most flattering for my shape.*

216

it makes a really great look. I also love to pair a stripy T-shirt with white jeans during the summer – this looks stunning with bright colours like red, pink and turquoise.

## Leather trousers

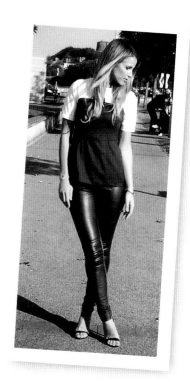

These might seem like an adventurous item to have in your wardrobe, but you'd be surprised how versatile they are, working equally well for daytime and night-time looks. It's definitely worth investing in a good-quality pair – my favourites cost me $500 around five years ago and they're still perfect. I wear them all the time. As with jeans, I normally buy a pair that are a little too small for me because they always stretch out. I tend to stick with classic black, as it's easier to match with other items in my wardrobe, but I also have a red pair for when I'm in the mood for something different. If leather trousers seem a bit too far outside your comfort zone, I would suggest trying wet-look leggings – you can pick up a pair fairly cheaply from Topshop or ASOS – to dip your toe in the water. I like to wear my trousers with a white T-shirt or cosy jumper for daytime and cute top and blazer for evenings out.

## Blazer

This jacket style works really well with my everyday leather trousers and T-shirt look, dressing it up really nicely, so I have quite a few in my wardrobe. I tend to stick with classic black and prefer a loose, over-sized style. But a short, fitted style is nice to throw on over dresses and with jeans.

## Bomber jackets

Bombers are back and there are so many gorgeous styles. A plain, simple one is a nice alternative to a leather jacket during the warm summer months, but there are also fantastic patterned and embroidered ones that add a nice touch to a basic outfit. I have two in my wardrobe at the moment, in wine and khaki.

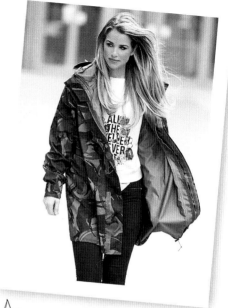

## Khaki coat

I think khaki is a great colour – it goes with absolutely everything, but is a nice alternative to black – and suggests a really casual style.

## Army coat

Tomboy alert! I have a few different styles and get lots of wear out of them – and an army coat is a festival staple for me.

*An army coat is a festival staple.*

## Mac

These are timeless. Burberry is famous for their beige macs, but I love my Aquascutum navy one. They are great for spring, as they're not too heavy and keep the inevitable rain off.

## Wool jumper

I divide most of my time between England and Ireland, neither of which are very warm, so I always have a new wool jumper ready to go.

## Hoodie

This is probably my tomboy side coming out again, but I have a lot of hoodies and wear them all the time. I love them under a leather jacket with some skinny jeans.

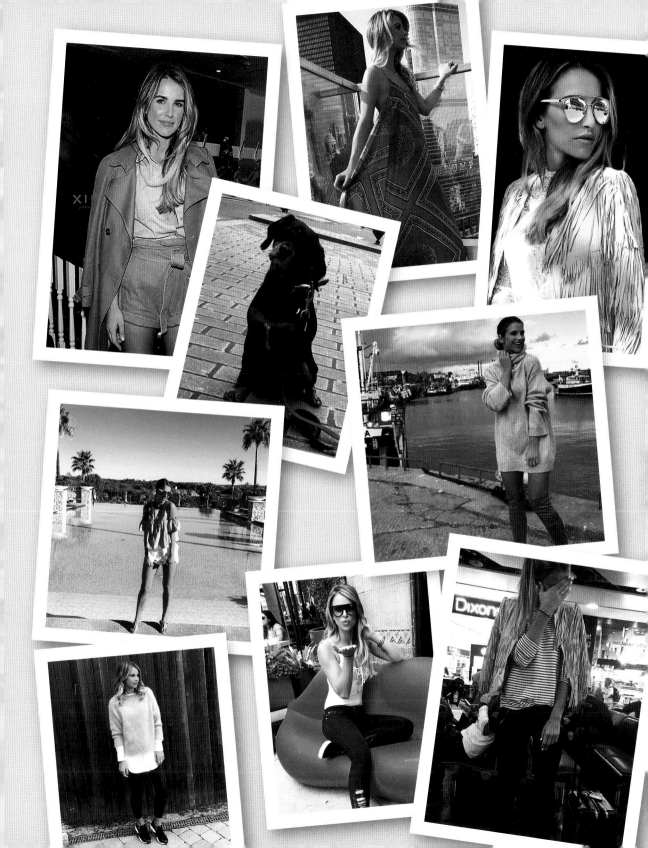

## LBD

Everyone should have a reliable black dress in their wardrobe that makes them feel like a million dollars.

# Completing an Outfit

## Hats

They can hide you from the world when you feel rough, but can also make any outfit instantly cooler. I wear a wool beanie on chilled-out days (a great way of hiding greasy hair too).

## Shoes

Shoes are one of life's great pleasures and a simple change of shoe can transform an outfit! I love runners and heels equally, so I have a lot of footwear.

### Runners/trainers

I'm a huge fan of runners, as I just can't deal with heels every day of the week. I think they can be worn with any outfit – I pair mine with dresses just as often as I do with jeans – and there are so many cool pairs out there. I tend to stick with classic white, but I also have a couple of coloured and metallic pairs for when I feel like introducing a pop of colour into

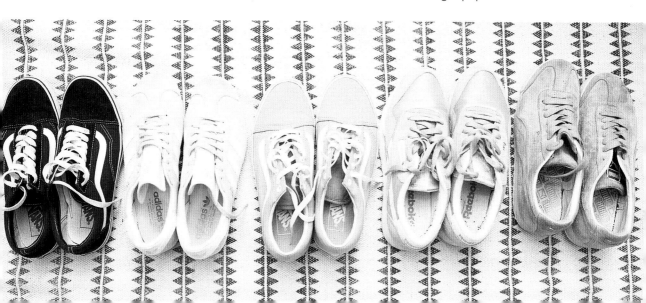

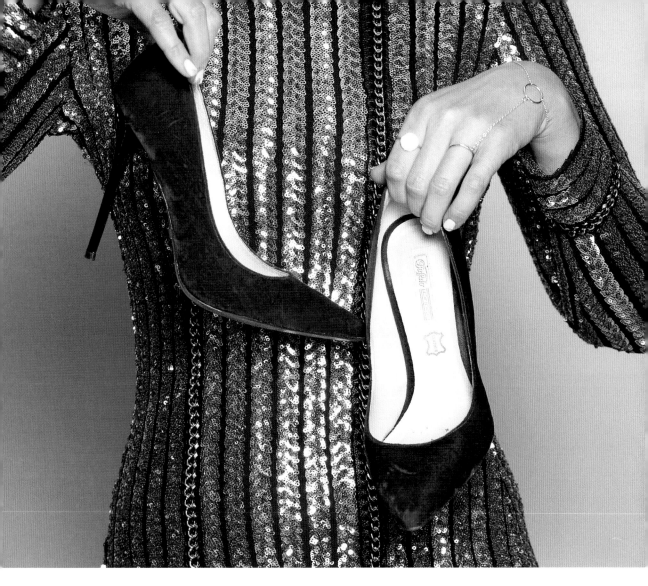

my outfit. Adidas Superstars have made a big comeback and are my go-to brand. I love a good pair of Vans too – they come in plenty of different designs – and I have a lot of Nike trainers and Asics for working out.

## Heels

Even though I'm tall, I love heels because I think they really lengthen your legs and make them appear slimmer. I don't think it's necessary to buy expensive heels – my collection is mostly high-street brands (it's the same when it comes to clothes) and my favourites are Office own brand and River Island. I must admit, though, that I do have a soft spot for shoes by Louboutin, Sophia Webster and Jimmy Choo. Usually I buy myself a pair by one of these designers as a present for my birthday or if I've been working really hard! But, when I consider cost per wear, they're a worthwhile investment because I wear them to death.

I always try on shoes before I buy them, because there is nothing worse than having a pair of heels that hurt – and they can really damage your feet. Comfort is important – we've all bought heels that don't fit quite right or offer enough support, and they gather dust in the wardrobe because we can't bear to wear them out! You shouldn't have to stretch out a pair of heels. It's also good to see if you can walk properly in them – it can look and feel very awkward if you can't, and wearing heels should give you confidence, not take it away.

I have four staple pairs that go with everything: two pairs of courts – one in nude and one in black – which I mostly wear during the winter; then, for summertime, I switch to strappy styles – I have a pair in beige and one in black.

## Bags

My bag collection is not quite as big as my shoe collection, but it's getting there! You do need different bags for different occasions, so it's important to have a lot – that's what I tell myself, anyway! But if you want to keep your own collection small, I would recommend getting both clutch bags and tote/day bags in basic styles and colours. I mostly use clutch bags for events and evenings out, but make sure not to get too small a size (otherwise you'll have trouble fitting anything other than your phone in there!). And, as with my heels, I mostly use black- and nude-

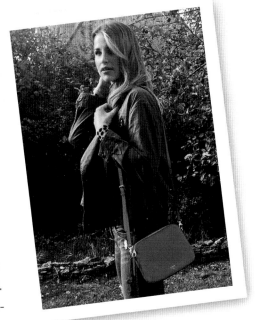

The bigger the bag, the more stuff you end up putting in it!

coloured styles, as they go with pretty much everything.

I don't really need to carry much about with me during the day, but I still always manage to fill up my large tote bags. The bigger the bag, the more stuff you end up putting in it! Again, I get most wear out of the styles I own in grey, black and nude/beige – but I do like colour sometimes too. At the moment, I own a couple of designer bags but have my eye on a few for my next purchase. At the top of my list is Givenchy!

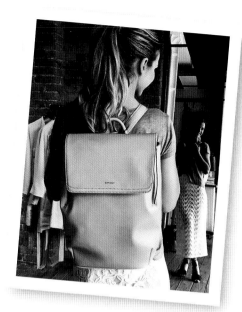

## Jewellery

Though I wear the occasional silver piece, I am definitely a gold girl. I buy a lot of accessories on the high street, but I've recently started to invest in gold-plated or gold pieces – ones I really love and that I want to have in my jewellery box for longer than high-street pieces usually last. And I really like building my collection, as it's such an easy way of changing up my basic outfits – I have pieces from fifteen years ago that I still wear now.

I used to love costume jewellery but, at the moment, I prefer more dainty pieces.

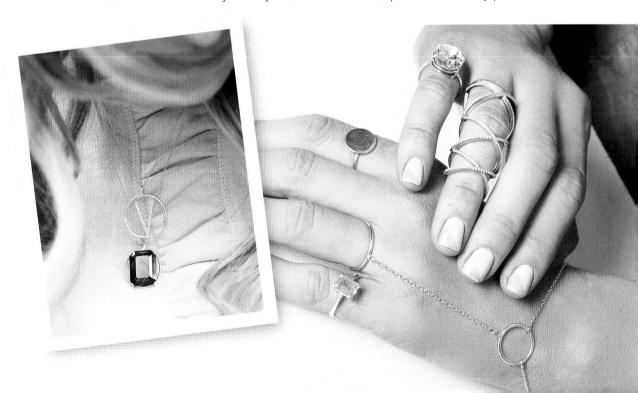

## Sunglasses

I think I would be slightly embarrassed if anyone was to count how many pairs of sunglasses I own. My collection is a little bit out of control, ranging from designer to high street to a pair I bought for $5 from a corner stall in New York. Sunglasses can make a look. If I wear an all-black outfit, I like to wear a quirky pair of shades to brighten it up a little and add a bit of personality. And I love the ability to hide behind shades – I mean, what would we do without them on a hangover day?

## Belts

I am always on the hunt for a good belt. It breaks up an outfit and makes you look slimmer too. Vintage shops are great places to look for cool styles. And, being tall, it's one of the few things that actually fits me when I go in.

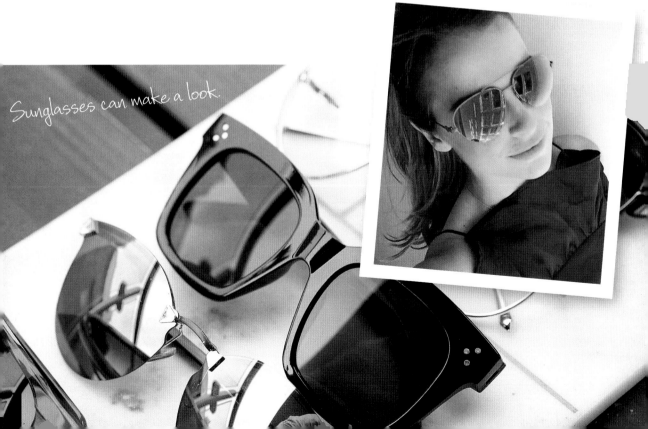

*Sunglasses can make a look.*

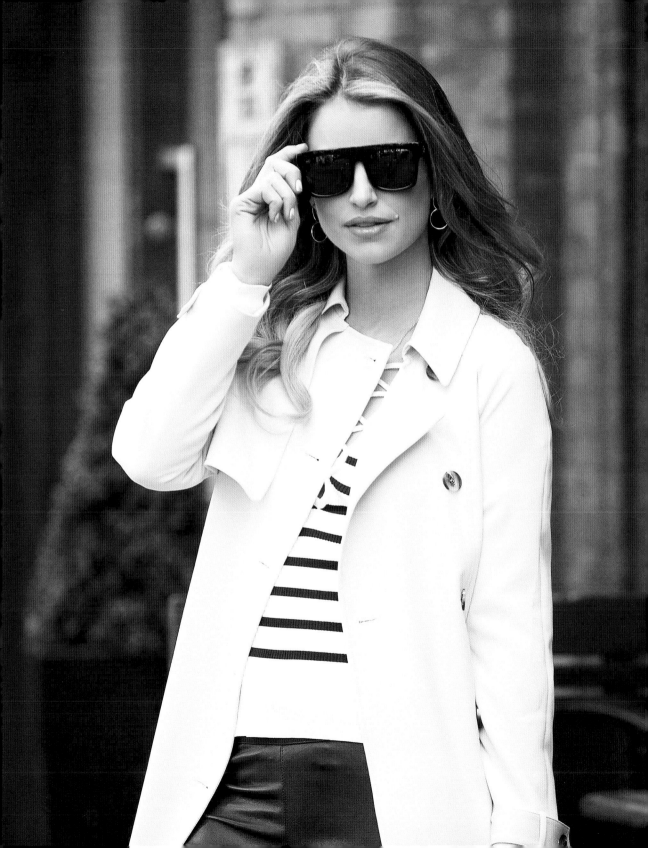

# Closet Clear-out

I think this is my friends' favourite thing for me to do – when I do a big clear-out, they definitely benefit!

Someone once told me that we wear 20 per cent of our clothes 80 per cent of the time – and I'm definitely guilty of having my wardrobe favourites that I stick to. I like to go through all my clothes every three months and get rid of things I know I'll never wear again, making room for all the new clothes I've acquired. We all have so many pieces in our wardrobes that we never wear, so be ruthless when you do a clear-out.

The easiest way is to start with each group of clothing items. I do tops first, then move on to jeans and keep going like that until I'm done. Anything that you haven't worn in ages (my personal rule is six months) can go, because you'll just leave it sitting there for another six months if you don't. Obviously, you will need to make an exception when it comes to occasion-wear, as you may not have had an opportunity to wear it recently. When I'm getting rid of designer pieces, I give them to a company that sells on designer items, so it's a good way to make money for more clothes! I offer all the other stuff I'm clearing out to my friends – I might have become bored with something or realised that it doesn't really suit me, but it might be the perfect addition to one of their wardrobes. And then what they don't take goes straight to the charity shop. Having a super-organised wardrobe makes life so much easier too – once I realise I have more pairs of blue jeans than I could possibly need, it makes it easier to talk myself out of buying yet another pair when I'm out shopping. Yet, I might spot that a simple black blazer would work well with lots of items I'm keeping, so I'll bear that in mind when I'm indulging in my next bout of retail therapy.

I think I get my ruthless clearing habits from my mom. I steal her clothes a lot, but I often look back at pictures of her from twenty years ago – when she was rocking a Sienna Miller, boho vibe – and ask her, fingers crossed, if she still has any of those pieces. And I'm always disappointed when she tells me that she's thrown them away. Such a shame, as I'm really crushing on that look right now.

Fashion to me is a big loop that keeps going around and around. I think everything comes in and out of fashion over the years, so it can be hard to throw things away because I know at some stage it will come back into fashion.

# Different Looks for Different Occasions

## The big night out

I love getting dressed up for a big night out. I spend a lot of my time in casual clothes and rock a tomboy style most days, but my going-out looks are always very girly.

There's nothing better than getting ready to go out with friends. I usually have a few of the girls over to my place and we'll have a couple of drinks and put on some music to get us in the mood for hitting the town.

I think a short dress is perfect for a night out. I rub Charlotte Tilbury Supermodel Body Shimmer down the front and back of my legs after my shower – it's a great body highlighter and will make your legs look slimmer. If you don't like wearing short dresses or skirts, a pair of skinny jeans and cute top is a winner for a night out too.

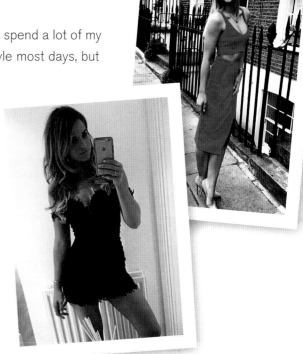

*I spend a lot of my time in casual clothes but my going-out looks are always very girly.*

## Dinner with friends

I go for dinner with my friends as often as I can – food is one of the best things in life and I love trying new restaurants. A lot of my friends have more standard Monday to Friday, nine-to-five work schedules, so I catch up with them over dinner in the evening all the time.

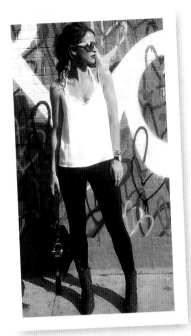

I don't like to go overboard when dressing for this kind of evening out, but I always like to look nice and like I've made an effort – just not too much of an effort. Jeans or leather trousers are my usual choices, as they're casual, but when you wear them with killer heels you instantly have a polished look. But make sure that you're comfortable in whatever it is you're wearing – you don't want to be put off ordering dessert by a too-tight waistband.

When it comes to the dressy top I wear to match, I would wear a crop top or something from AQ/AQ – they do lovely structured ones that instantly dress up an outfit.

I finish the look with a really nice coat or jacket, nothing too heavy, a cute bag and some simple gold jewellery. I think a wardrobe staple is a leather jacket and I would usually wear one of mine on a night out.

*Jeans or leather trousers are my usual choices, as they're casual.*

## First date

I don't usually do romantic dinner dates until I have known someone a while. But when I find myself with one in the diary, I like a look that's flirty but not too dressed up. I might go for a basic structured top and jeans with a killer heel – but make the outfit look super cool with a leopard-print coat.

## Third date

Once I've got to know the person I'm seeing a bit better – and I know that I like spending time with them – I might dress to

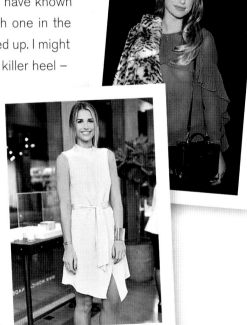

impress a little more. I would probably wear a cute dress – one that is over the knee, tight on top and looser around the legs. I would throw a simple blazer over this kind of look.

## Saturday brunch

It's all about comfort, especially if I'm feeling tired after a long week. I'll throw on my favourite pair of blue jeans, a plain T-shirt and a blazer, adding a pair of sunglasses and a beanie.

## Sunday afternoon in the pub

Relaxing on a Sunday afternoon is all about being cosy. In winter, I'd usually be found wearing a woolly jumper – my favourite right now is a pink H&M one that I sometimes

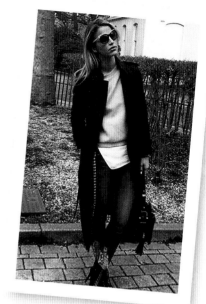

*It's all about comfort.*

wear as a dress with trainers, which is equally comfortable. If it's cold out, I'll wear it with leather trousers. In summer I'd usually go with a plain T-shirt, blazer and jeans or shorts if the weather was good.

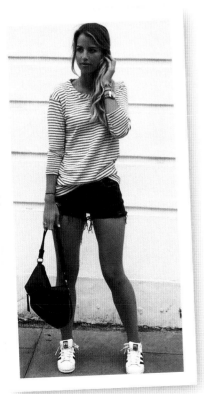

## Cheat day outfit

Sometimes I end up staying in my PJs all day – but I try not to do that too often! Usually I'm wearing a soft hoodie, tracksuit pants, a concert T-shirt and a fluffy pair of slippers. I can be quite hungover on my cheat day – I think it's best to have your cheat day after a night out, as you always crave bad food anyway. I love Lucy Nagle – she's an Irish designer who makes the softest cashmere pieces – and if I'm hungover I wear my Lucy Nagle cashmere tracksuit. When you're hungover, being wrapped in cashmere makes everything better!

229

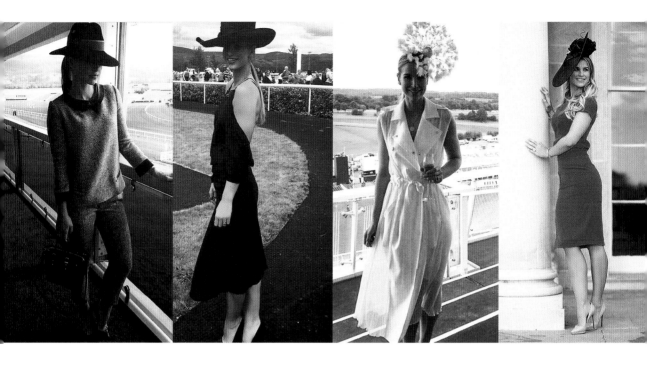

# The Big Events

## Racing fashion

I am a huge fan of going to the races and am lucky enough to have been asked to judge the Ladies Day fashion. The prizes for the winner are always amazing, so make sure to enter any time you find yourself at the races on Ladies Day. I have seen so many gorgeous outfits, but also a lot that are more suited to a Saturday night out, which is a big no-no for me.

My top tip for dressing for the races is quite simple: dress like you're going to meet your boyfriend's parents for the first time. Going to the races requires quite a conservative dress sense, so a beautiful dress below the knee is always appropriate.

I like to choose my outfit first and then I match my shoes, bag and hat. A hat or headpiece is vital – it's the one event where it's necessary to wear one. I sometimes see women with the most gorgeous outfits, but when they aren't wearing a hat, their outfit looks unfinished.

I would like to say wear comfortable shoes, given that it's a long day and involves walking on uneven ground, but I don't always stick to that rule myself – heels are the way to go to complete a dressy ensemble like this.

## Wedding looks

I think people find it hard to dress for a wedding. Though we all love to be a part of the special days of our loved ones, buying an outfit for a wedding can be expensive, especially when you factor in accessories to match. It's also tricky to find an outfit that works equally well for the ceremony and evening celebrations and is comfortable enough for all-day wear – also, you want to look good but not so good that you'll take any attention away from the bride!

Anything white is definitely out: the bride is the only person allowed to wear white. More generally, I tend to keep to the rules I use when I'm dressing for the races – anything too revealing won't work at all. I think a three-quarter-length dress is perfect.

For a summer wedding, I think bright colours work well, but for a winter wedding, I would be more inclined to wear muted tones – though I think that's just winter dressing in general.

I would wear a dress with tights underneath and a nice coat over my outfit. I always wear really comfortable shoes because you end up standing for a big portion of the day. You can get heel caps that go over stilettos so if you're outside on the grass it makes it a lot easier to walk and you won't sink into the mud.

I dress up my outfits with matching accessories and team my look with a clutch handbag.

I team my look with a clutch handbag.

## The black-tie event

For those extra-special events, which usually only come along once or twice a year, we don't want to look anything but amazing! I like to go all out for events like this and I'm in the lucky position of being able to borrow amazing dresses for just one night. But renting a dress is a great option to keep in mind – it's something I also do a lot. Most stores that offer rentals have gorgeous designer dresses that you can rent at a fraction of the retail price and you can have them fitted as well.

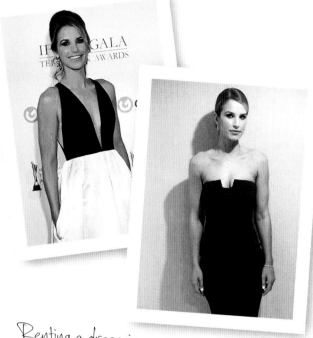

*Renting a dress is a great option to keep in mind.*

# Packing

Packing is the bane of my life. But because I spend most of the time living out of a suitcase, I have become something of a reluctant packing expert.

If I'm going away for a weekend, I only take hand luggage – a roomy tote bag or helpfully named 'weekender' bag should give you all the room you need. It's tempting to take lots of things with you, but you really don't need to pack much, and being organised will make a big difference. I plan outfits for the time I'm away and reuse pieces like jeans and jackets (which are bulky to pack). And you can put socks and underwear into shoes to save space but you shouldn't need to if you organise well.

Hotels always have hairdryers, so there is no need to pack one. I keep a small clear bag with shampoo and conditioner, cleanser, moisturiser and toothpaste in my house so it's always ready to go. You can buy little pots in chemists that are the right size to get through security checks at an airport.

# Packing for a short city break

I decided in 2016 that I needed to start seeing more places, and I'm enjoying visiting different cities. Usually, a city break is quite short, so you can get away with just taking cabin baggage. Here is what I would pack for a two-night city break:

* **1 pair of blue jeans:** when you're short on space, it's best to take items that can be used for multiple outfits. A basic pair of blue jeans can be worn for a casual look during the day and a dressy look in the evening.

* **1 pair of black leather pants:** as with the jeans, these can be casual or dressy. If leather pants aren't for you, you might try wet-look leggings or even a cool pair of black jeans.

* **2 plain T-shirts/casual tops:** perfect for during the day.

* **2 evening tops:** I usually go for a silky camisole and a sparkly top.

* **1 pair of heels**

* **1 pair of trainers:** I usually wear these to the airport.

* **2 jumpers:** these obviously depend on where you're going and at what time of year. But, especially when it comes to springtime or late autumn, you never really know what the weather will be like so it's best to be prepared.

* **1 little black dress:** just in case you end up going somewhere quite fancy.

* **1 blazer:** these are easily packed, don't take up too much room and go well with night-time looks.

* **Underwear and socks**

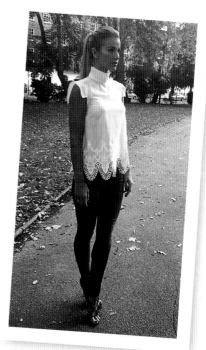

*A basic pair of blue jeans can be worn for a casual look during the day and a dressy look in the evening.*

233

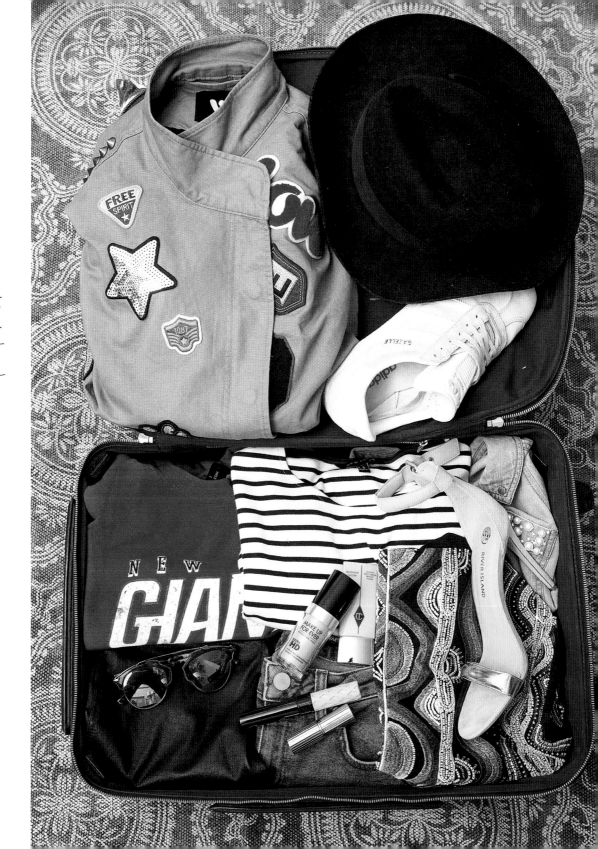

What I pack for a two-night city break

* **1 pair of leggings and 2 gym tops:** I know this sounds boring, but I like to maintain my training regime even when I'm away.

* **1 warm coat:** choose one that is versatile enough to be worn during the day and in the evening. You can wear this to the airport so it doesn't take up space in your bag.

* **Ready-to-go toiletries bag**

## Packing for a two-week sun holiday

Just writing this is making me think of my next sun holiday – I can't wait! I usually pack too much, but over the years I have learned to minimise the amount I bring to include only the essentials – it also means that I can do a little shopping while I'm away.

I spend a lot of time at the beach and, after years of packing lots of pairs of shorts and not wearing most of them, I now only bring dresses for the beach, as they're so easy to throw on over my bikini. Shorts get wet and uncomfortable at the beach but a loose dress is always a winner.

I buy my sun cream in the airport – they always have good deals and it means I don't add weight to my already heavy bag. And I often make use of washing services in the hotels and apartments I'm staying in, so it means I can re-wear a lot of what I bring.

Here's what I would bring for a two-week holiday:

* **10 bikinis:** I know I bring too many, but I like to mix it up and they're small and easy to pack.

* **4–5 beach dresses:** I wear these every day, so I bring quite a few in case some end up getting dirty.

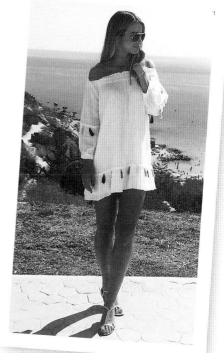

*I only bring dresses to the beach as they're easy to throw over my bikini.*

235

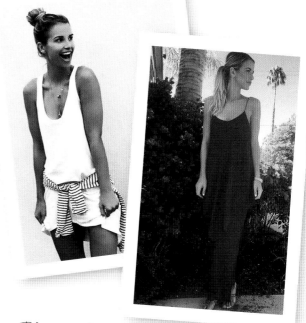

* **2 pairs of denim cut-off shorts, one black and one blue:** though I don't wear them on the beach, these look great over a swimsuit during the day, if you're going out for lunch, or in the evening with a nice flowy top.

* **2 miniskirts**

* **2 short dresses**

* **4–5 daytime tops:** if I'm not at the beach, I'll be wandering around in a top and shorts. Usually I keep it pretty simple and bring T-shirts or camisoles. It's a good idea to include a long-sleeved T-shirt or cardigan, just in case the evening is cold or you need to cover up after getting a bit too much sun.

*It's a good idea to include a long-sleeved t-shirt or cardigan in case the evening is cold.*

* **1 evening top**

* **2 maxi dresses:** these work well for day and night looks. I like to bring one simple white one and another in a colour or print.

* **2 pairs of sandals:** I bring a beige pair and a black pair so they go with everything.

* **1 pair of flip-flops:** perfect for hanging out around the pool and at the beach.

* **2 pairs of heels:** again, I would bring a black and a nude sandal so they will go with everything.

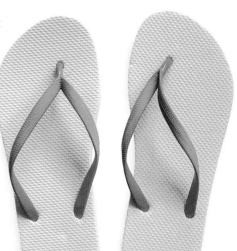

What I pack for a two-week sun holiday.

* **Training gear:** I pack a few outfits, as I keep up my training routine on holiday.

* **4 pairs of sunglasses:** again this is excessive, but I like to have a lot of options, and I throw these in my hand luggage.

* **2 hats:** I wear hats every day on the beach to keep the sun off my face.

* **Underwear and socks**

* **Jewellery:** I always take quite a bit, as it's an easy way of dressing simple outfits up, but do carry these pieces in your hand luggage – they'll weigh too much in your check-in luggage.

* **Music:** I know this seems like an odd one, but when I'm away, I spend hours and hours listening to music – I always buy about six new albums before I go away to get me through those long days on the beach.

## Bikini tips

It's so important to get a bikini that fits well. I don't like them too tight on the bottoms, as it can often look like you have a little muffin top even if you don't! That goes for all clothes, but with bikinis, there's not much material to hide areas you usually would, and you definitely don't want to feel self-conscious when you're supposed to be enjoying your holiday.

I don't have huge boobs (unfortunately!) so I don't need an underwire bikini top, but I do like them with a little bit of padding. If you do need that extra bit of support, it's a good idea to visit a store that sells lingerie as well, because the staff will be able to fit you for a bikini the same way they would for a bra.

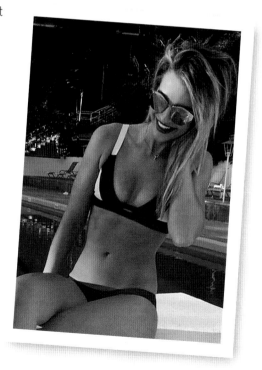

I used to go a size up in bikinis so they wouldn't be super tight, but a bikini designer told me that this was not the way to go – you should stick to your size, as they always loosen up a bit when you wear them. It's very important to try on a few bikinis, in different styles, before buying. There are so many styles out there now to suit all body shapes – it's definitely worth having a look around and investing in a good swimsuit or bikini. Nobody has the perfect body so just find a suit that flatters yours.

Bikinis only last a couple of years, but if you wash them when you're away, they can last a little bit longer – chlorine can ruin them so always rinse them after you've been in the pool.

# Festivals

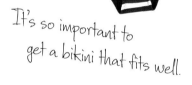

It's so important to get a bikini that fits well.

## Festival dressing

I love going to festivals. Sometimes I don't end up seeing that many acts, but I love hanging out, having drinks with my friends and getting to meet new people. Festivals have a different atmosphere to anything else – there's such a sense of fun and freedom. I went to Electric Picnic one year and only saw three acts all weekend – that was bad even for me, but I had such a good time.

Festival fashion is my favourite: you can wear whatever you like and get away with it. I don't really do the whole floral headband thing, but I do sometimes wear a hat for day two when my hair is no longer looking on fleek!

I always wear shorts or a dress to a festival, regardless of the weather, because they're comfy (the sun often comes out). Whatever you wear, make sure you feel comfortable and always bring layers because it can get seriously cold. I bring a big jumper for when it gets cold and a jacket for the inevitable rain showers.

Never wear heels to a festival – you'll be running around in a field all day so runners or wellies are essential.

# Festival hacks

## Tent

I don't camp at festivals anymore but over the years I've learned a few tips. First, buy a pop-up tent because the last thing you want to do is spend ages pitching your tent. With a pop-up, all you need to do is take it out of the bag and it does all the work for you!

You should also bring something like an old scarf that will enable you to identify your tent easily. I always bring a lock for my tent and give a spare key to whoever I am with.

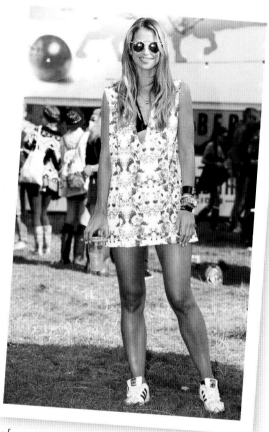

Bring a lilo or yoga mat to put on the floor of your tent, and you can get a little blow-up pillow too for extra comfort. They'll be easy to carry and won't take up a lot of space. And don't forget your sleeping bag.

## Clothes

You will always need more clothes than you think, so pack well. For sleeping I would always bring thermals and a tracksuit – you can also wear the tracksuit home on your last day when everything else is covered in mud. Pack your festival looks for each day and then, on top of that, bring extra jumpers. I always pack loads of socks, two pairs of trainers and my wellies. A light raincoat you can fold up into your handbag is also essential for those pesky showers we get in Ireland.

## Food

I get my meals from the stalls at the festival but I always have a little bit of food – crisps and chocolate usually – in my bag to keep me going in case I get really hungry. If you're camping, make sure you have a lot of water in your tent – you can buy it at the stalls in the festival site.

## Money

I always find the ATMs super busy at festivals so get there early and get your money for the day. Don't carry too much with you in case you lose it – and be careful with your bag too. The best option for a festival is a cross-body bag so you can keep a proper eye on it.

## Phone charger

There are so many portable chargers available these days and they aren't expensive so make sure you bring a few away with you. The last thing you want is to get separated from your friends when your phone battery is about to die.

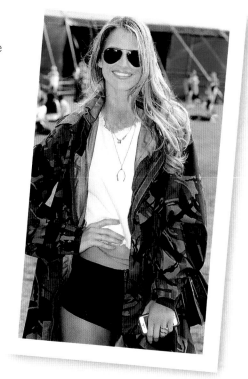

## Set times

Print the set times off before the festival so you always know when people are playing – there is less likelihood of missing your favourite bands this way.

## Chemist

I like to bring my own version of a pharmacy away with me – three days' drinking is tough on anyone and if you hit it hard you will need all of these: painkillers, anti-nausea tablets, Berocca and Dioralyte.

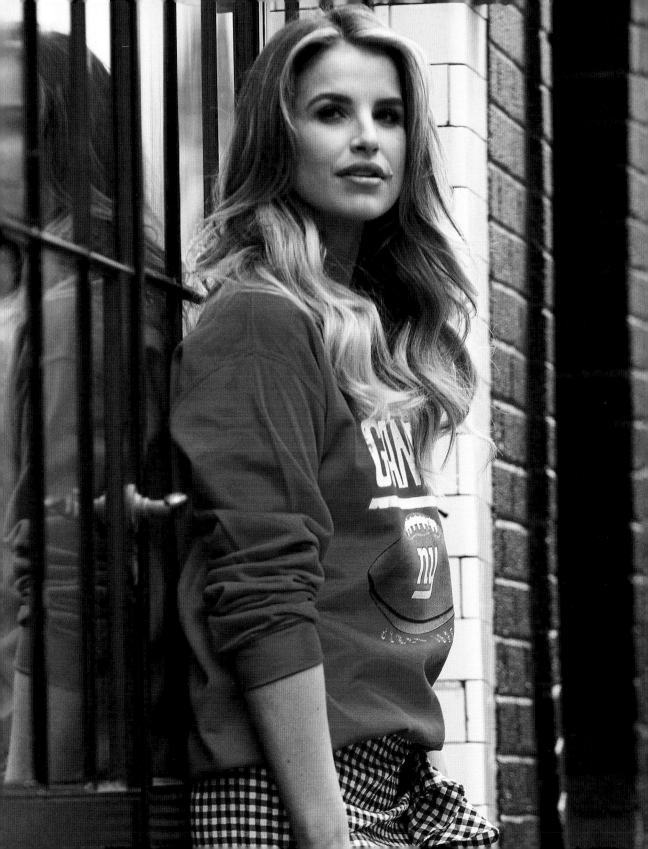

# Life hacks

I'm often asked how I got into the career I have so I wanted to take this opportunity to offer an answer. I'm so lucky to be doing my dream job – and I suppose some parts of it are unusual in comparison to other professions – but when it comes down to it, what I do has a lot in common with any other job, and progression and achievement happen in the same way.

First, it takes a lot of focus, ambition and hard work. When I realised that working as a model and in the media was what I wanted to do, I knew that it was going to be difficult to achieve and would involve a lot of hard graft and disappointment. And difficult conversations with my parents! My advice would be to work as hard as you can, to make the most out of every opportunity that comes your way and try not to take any setbacks to heart. I've always tried to learn as much as I can from mistakes and disappointments. Though it's not always seen as such, I think ambition is a great quality in a person. And it's vital if you want to achieve your dreams.

My job isn't as glamorous as it looks. Don't get me wrong – it can be lots of fun! But I don't have as much time off as I would like – I usually end up with one day off a week rather than two but, thankfully, I really enjoy my job and having lots on the go at any given time. And sometimes you need to be willing to make some sacrifices if you want to succeed, especially in the media industry, which so many people want to work in. It can make finding time to see friends and family very difficult, but sometimes it's about recognising that you have to make time for what's important – so I often get up earlier and go to bed later to fit everything in.

You should try to think outside the box: what is going to make you different from everyone else? I am always writing notes in my phone for different ideas for TV shows or columns – anything that comes to my mind gets written down, so I can expand on the idea when I get home.

Stay focused too – there is always a lot of disappointment in any career, particularly at the start, but you have to stay focused on what you want and don't stop until you get it. I'm a real girl's girl, and I like to see other people doing well. I've gone for jobs that I've really wanted and other girls have ended up getting them. Instead of getting myself down about it, I always just moved forward to the next thing. That job obviously wasn't right for me or meant for me, and there will be something even better around the corner.

Remember to always be nice in business because people never forget. You need to believe in yourself and be positive – this can be hard if you have setbacks, but if you put out positive energy you'll get it back in return. I don't like people who are willing to trample over someone else to further their career. I don't like nastiness and dishonesty – if you act like this, people always remember and you never know who you'll end up meeting in the future.

I always put myself out there: if I hear of a job I want, I make sure to at least get a meeting for it or make contact with someone in charge. If you don't try, you won't get, so always give it a go – even if you don't get it, at least you can say you tried.

Every year I write myself a list of goals instead of New Year's resolutions. When I have written them, I work my hardest towards achieving them during the year. The goals do have to be within reason – winning the lottery isn't a goal – but goals that are personal to you and that will help you with your career are worth working towards.

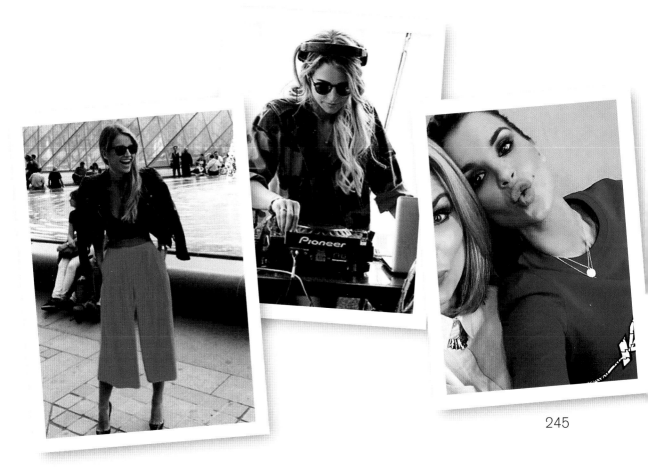

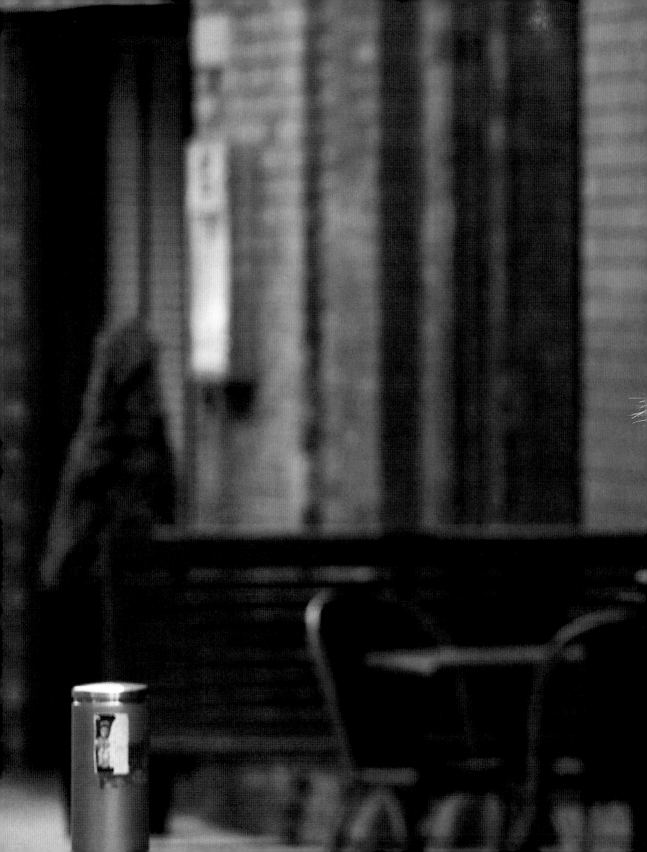

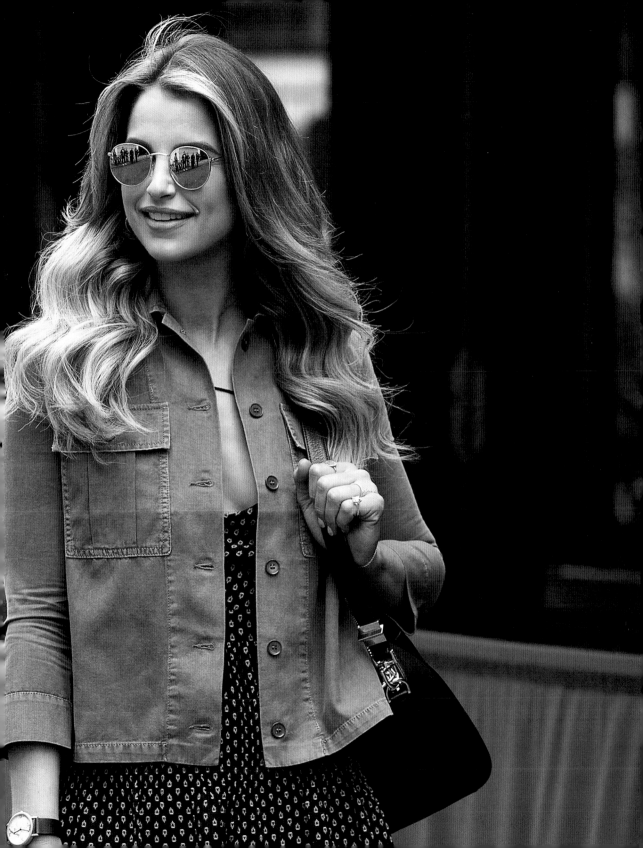

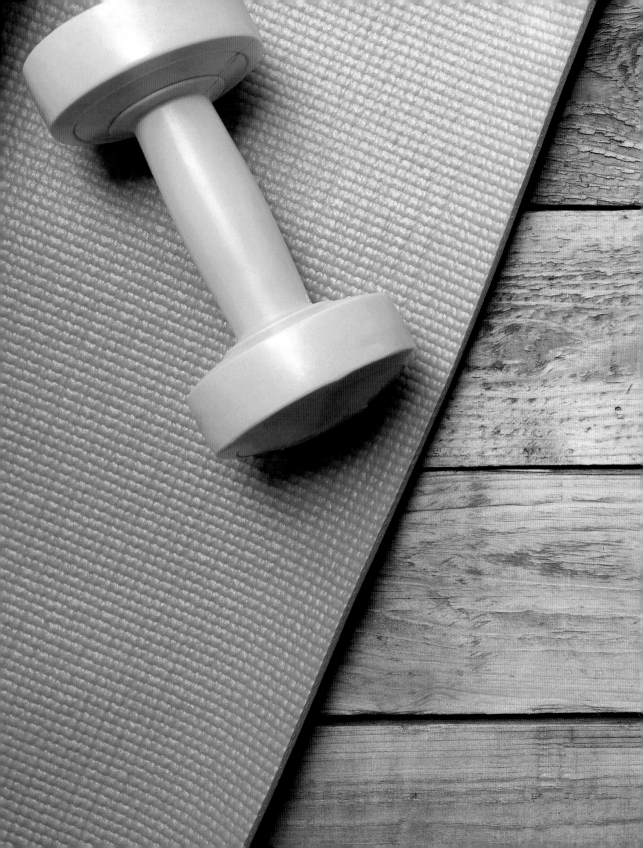

# More exercise routines

# Ollie Frost

Here are former professional rugby player's Ollie Frost's six exercises for total body conditioning and strength. Ollie currently works as a strength and conditioning coach. This workout should take about forty-five minutes. www.olliefrost.com

## Exercise 1: dumb-bell renegade row x 4 sets, 6–10 reps each side

This exercise will build both upper- and lower-body strength while engaging all your muscles in your back to maintain correct alignment. This will help develop strength at your abdomen.

1. Place two dumb-bells on the floor in front of you about shoulder-width apart.
2. Position yourself as though you are going to do a push-up but hold on to the dumb-bells. Ensure your body is straight and extended and that you are on your toes. This is your starting and finishing position. The dumb-bells will support your upper body. You may need to position your feet wide for support.
3. Bending your right arm at the elbow, lift one dumb-bell until it is roughly at your waist. You will have to retract your shoulder blade on the side you are working as you flex your elbow. Your left arm should be straight.
4. Lower the dumb-bell to the floor and then lift it in your left hand.

## Exercise 2: Spider-Man push-up x 4 sets, 8 reps each side

The Spider-Man push-up is a variation of the standard push-up – the difference is that it adds in hip flexion. It's named after Spider-Man, as the action resembles him climbing up a wall, but for us, it's just done on the floor. This exercise is excellent for improving hip flexibility and will increase total body strength.

1. Get into a traditional push-up position.
2. As you lower yourself towards the floor, bring your right knee to your right elbow, keeping it off the ground.

3. Press back up to the starting position.
4. Repeat, this time bringing your left knee to your left elbow.

### Exercise 3: dumb-bell thruster, 3 sets of 10 reps

The dumb-bell thruster is a challenging multi-joint exercise that targets the legs, shoulders and arms. It's a great total body exercise that will help burn fat and increase strength.

1. Stand with your feet shoulder-width apart, holding a dumb-bell in each hand but resting on your shoulders.
2. Squat down, ensuring your hips go below your knees, but keep your back straight.
3. Stand up and, as you do, straighten your arms, so you push the dumb-bells above your head.

### Exercise 4: V-up x 4 sets, 5–20 reps

Abdominal V-ups work both the upper and lower abdominal muscles at the same time. You don't need any equipment; ensure all technical points are looked at to maximise benefits.

1. Lie flat on the floor with your lower back and shoulders pressed into the ground and your arms extended behind your head with your palms facing the ceiling.
2. Keep your feet together and your toes pointed at the ceiling.
3. In one movement, lift your legs, keeping them straight, and raise your upper body from the floor. Reach for your toes with your hands. Engage and squeeze your abdominal muscles as you reach for your toes.
4. Slowly lower your body and legs back to the starting position.

### Exercise 5: plank push-up x 3 sets, 10–20 reps

This is a great abdominal exercise that will also challenge your upper body.

1.  Start in a plank position – this is similar to a normal push-up, but rest on your elbows. Your feet should be shoulder-width apart and your body should be straight.
2.  Press your body up to a push-up position, one arm at a time, and then lower yourself back down into the plank, one arm at a time.

### Exercise 6: dumb-bell split lunge x 4 sets, 8 reps for each leg

The dumb-bell split lunge is a variation on the squat that you can use to build strength and power in your legs and hips, particularly your quads (thigh muscles) and bum.

1.  Stand with your right leg in front of your left, holding a dumb-bell in each hand at your side.
2.  Bend the knee of your right leg to lower into a lunge until your thigh is parallel to the ground. Ensure your right knee is behind your toes.
3.  Extend your hip and knee to drive up to the start position.
4.  When you have finished your reps on your right leg, repeat with your left leg.

# Megan Farmer

I have had a lot of fantastic training sessions with Megan in the past, but she has now left personal training to study to be a midwife, which is a job I know she'll be brilliant at. She was nicknamed 'Mean Meg' by some of her clients, but personally I loved her no-nonsense approach – I know that she expected nothing less than 100 per cent from me during our sessions, and that pushed me to give my all.

## Workout 1

This workout should take forty minutes. Aim to do four circuits with as little rest as possible.

### Exercise 1: jumping lunges x 24 reps

See page 36.

### Exercise 2: Lie-down push-ups x 15 reps

1.  Lie flat on your tummy with your legs straight and open to about shoulder-width apart. Stretch your arms straight out ahead of you.
2.  Breathe in and place your hands flat on the ground beside your shoulders, tuck your toes under and push up into a full press-up.
3.  Gently lower your body back down to the ground as you breathe out.

### Exercise 3: hand-release burpees x 12 reps

1.  From a standing position, squat down, placing both hands on the floor, either side of your feet.
2.  Jump your feet back into a plank position.
3.  Lower your body to the ground and release your hands.

4. Place your hands back on the floor pushing back up into the full-body plank.
5. Jump your feet in and jump back up to a standing position.

### Exercise 4: single-leg tricep dips x 10 reps each side

1. Sit with your back to a bench (or chair or step – you can use anything like this as long as it is stable and secure to take your body weight).
2. Reaching back, put your hands onto the bench. They should be shoulder-width apart with your fingers facing forward and elbows pointing backwards with a slight bend in the elbow. Your legs should be extended out in front of you with a slight bend in the knee.
3. Hoist yourself up until your arms are nearly straight, but do not lock them.
4. Slowly lower your body until your shoulder joints are below your elbows.
5. Push back up again until your elbows are nearly straight.

### Exercise 5: box jumps x 20 reps (use a high/low step or a sturdy platform)

1. Stand in an upright position, with your feet shoulder-width apart, at a comfortable distance from the box.
2. Jump up and drop quickly into a quarter squat.
3. Extend your hips, swing your arms and push your feet through the floor to propel yourself onto the box.
4. Gently jump back off the box landing softly on your feet with your knees slightly bent.

# Workout 2: Abs

Do three rounds in total.

### Exercise 1: super crunch x 15 reps

1.  Lying flat on your back with legs fully extended and arms stretched over your head, bring your knees to your chest.
2.  Bring your arms over your head, lifting your head and shoulders up, and reach for your heels.
3.  Stretch back out into the starting position.
4.  Ensure you keep your tummy muscles engaged.

### Exercise 2: toe touch x 30 reps

1.  Lie down with your back flat to the floor.
2.  Raise your legs straight up in the air – ensure your tummy is tight.
3.  With straight arms, stretch up and reach for your toes with your fingertips, keeping your head and shoulders off the ground the whole time. This is like mini pulses.
4.  If your neck gets sore keep your hands at the back of your head.

### Exercise 3: bicycle crunches x 40 reps

1.  Lie on your back with your legs stretched out long and your hands at the back of your head.
2.  Lift your head and shoulders up and touch your right elbow off your left knee.
3.  At the same time, keep the opposite leg straight and a few inches off the floor.
4.  Alternate so your left elbow touches your right knee – keep alternating.
5.  Keep your tummy tight and make sure to keep your elbows back so that you are not straining your neck.

### Exercise 4: floor touches x 20 reps

1. Lie on your back. Ensure your back is flat on the floor and your tummy is nice and tight.
2. Bend your knees so they are open and hip-width apart and stretch your arms behind your head.
3. As you breathe out, bring your arms over your head, sitting up all the way and tipping in between your feet.
4. Breathe in slowly as you lower yourself back to the starting position.
5. Make sure to do this exercise slowly – do not bang your back on the return to the starting position.

# Workout 3

For this workout, you'll need two 2.5kg dumb-bells and a skipping rope. Do five rounds with as little rest as possible.

### Exercise 1: squat jump x 30 reps

1. Stand with your feet shoulder-width apart.
2. Start by doing a regular squat, then engage your core and jump up explosively.
3. As you land, lower your body back into the squat position.
4. Go straight into the next jump.

### Exercise 2: plank get-up x 15 reps

1. Start in a full plank position – on your hands and feet, head pushed over your shoulders, tummy tight and feet open, hip-width apart, ensuring that your hips stay still.
2. Breathe in, lower your hands down onto your elbows, then breathe out and come back up onto your hands. Ensure your tummy stays tight and hips remain still and in position and your elbows stay in line with your shoulders.

### Exercise 3: fast skip x 45 seconds

Standing in an upright position, skip as fast as you can. Remember to stay tall and keep your core strong.

### Exercise 4: lat raise x 15 reps

1. Stand tall with your feet hip-width apart and shoulders back.
2. Hold one 2.5kg dumb-bell in each hand, with hands by your sides.
3. As you breathe out, slowly raise both weights at the same time as high as your shoulders.
4. Pause for two seconds.
5. Breathing in very slowly, lower the weights back down by your sides.

### Exercise 5: tuck jump x 15 reps

1. Stand upright with your hands out in front of you at chest height.
2. Rapidly dip down into a quarter squat and immediately explode up, bringing your knees towards your chest. Try to touch your hands with your knees.
3. Land softly on your feet and ensure you keep your knees slightly bent.

# Acknowledgements

I'd like to thank all the people who helped in the production of this book:

**Photography:** Evan Doherty   www.thisisevan.com   @evandoherty   EvanDohertyStudio

**Stylist:** Corina Gaffey   www.corinagaffey.com   @corinagaffey   corinagaffey

**Stylist Assistant:** Eva Witter   @evawitter

**Make-Up:** Sarah Keary   www.sarahkeary.ie   @sarah_keary   sarahkearymakeup; Grainne Duffy   @GDuffystyle

**Hair:** Matthew Feeney   @glamfeeney   glamfeeney

**Exercise:** Erica Brennan, from The Gym Howth   www.thegymhowth.com   @thegymhowth; Maya Saffron, based at Virgin Active in London   mayasaffronhan; Ollie Frost www.olliefrost.com;   @Ollie_frost;   Megan Farmer   Meganfarmer21

**Recipes:** Dr Tara Coletta   taracoletta   And thanks to Sarah for the cocktail tips!

**Beauty:**
Kristina Kelly from the Renaissance Clinic in Howth   www.renaissanceclinic.ie

Nilam Patel, founder of beauty brand High Definition   @eyebrowqueen   @thebrowqueen

Ashley O'Rourke: www.ashleyorourke.com   @makeupashley   makeupbyashleyorourke

Rebecca Todd:   @rtoddmakeup   rebeccatoddmua

**Nails:** Tropical Popical   @tropicalpopical   tropicalpopical

**Tower Jewellers:** towerjewellers

**Illustrations:** Ciara Kenny   @Ciaraioch

**Fitness Location:** FLYEFit Gym, George's Street

Any errors that occur by accident in any of the exercise regimes, recipes or beauty advice are mine!

Thanks to my publishers Hachette Ireland and Katie Phillips and Katie French from KPPR.

To Louisa and Megan from Money Management Agency: I don't know how I haven't driven you two mad yet but you have been so brilliant throughout this entire book. You are both powerhouses and without you I would have struggled.

A special thanks to my very best friend and sister, Amber. I have always idolised you and I think you are one of the greatest people I know. Thank you for always being there for me.

My aunt and godmother Naomi who is my mom in Ireland! Naomi, you are always full of help and advice and I appreciate all of it.

My brother Frederick and Emma, your beautiful wife: there's nothing I love to do more when I get home than come and spend time with you two and Jeaniebops. Alexander, my little brother who I used as my real life doll as soon as you were born. There's nothing I love more than a text from you and I am so looking forward to you moving back to this side of the world. You always lift my spirits and stick up for me and I adore you for that.

Neil, my stepdad, but who is really a second dad to me: you have instilled my work ethic in me and without you, I doubt I would have achieved everything I have.

I don't want to name friends separately as I am lucky to have such a brilliant group of friends and there are way too many to mention but you all know who you are. My friends are like family to me and I feel incredibly lucky to have all of you in my life.

To my love, Spencer: thank you for helping me along this journey. I know there were times I let the workload get on top of me but you were always there to make me smile.

# Image credits

**Author's collection:** xi, 2, 3, 6, 7, 8, 11, 13, 15, 16, 17, 21, 26, 27, 143, 148, 156, 161 (above), 162, 166, 167, 170, 173 (above), 179 (below), 187, 189, 194, 196, 204, 207, 208 (above), 208 (middle), 210, 211, 214, 216 (below), 217, 218, 219, 222, 223 (above), 224 (inset), 227, 228, 229, 230, 231 (above), 232, 233, 235, 236 (above), 238, 240, 241, 245.

**Ciara Kenny (illustrations):** 35-37, 39, 40-43.

**Evan Doherty:** ii, vi-vii, viii, xii, 4, 23, 24, 33, 38, 48, 53, 56-57, 59, 60, 63 (above), 64, 68, 70, 118, 141, 145, 146, 151, 155, 159, 169, 173 (below), 175, 181, 188, 191, 197, 200, 203, 208 (below), 209, 212, 220, 221, 223 (below), 224 (below), 225, 234, 237, 242, 246-247.

**iStock:** 31/clubfoot, 66/4kodiak, 80/Rimma_Bondarenko, 90/AnthiaCumming, 108/melgfg, 119/Juanmonino, 140 & 142/Avosb, 157 (above)/PLAINVIEW, 157 (below)/imagehub88, 161 (below)/sdominick, 163/GrLb71, 177/fotografixx, 178/cc-stock, 179 (above)/dolgachov, 231 (below left)/zoranm, 231 (below right)/penguenstok, 248-249/Tatomm.

**Shutterstock.com:** 28/ronstik, 30/Tamas Ambrits, 55/verca, 63(below)/Anastasia Izofatova, 65/VICUSCHKA, 67/Tobik, 73/gephoto, 74/Irina Meliukh, 77/Brent Hofacker, 79/AnjelikaGr, 83/stockforlife, 84/casanisa, 87/Gayvoronskaya_Yana, 89/mpessaris, 93/naito29, 95/Vlasovalana, 97/fired, 99/Goskova Tatiana, 101/Bartosz Luczak, 102/Ildi Papp, 105/Timolina, 107/MariaKovaleva, 111/svariophoto, 112/Tiramisu Studio, 115/Ruslan Mitin, 116/bonchan, 117/Linda Hughes, 121/vm2002, 122/Anna_Pustynnikova, 125/Larisa Blinova, 126/Alexander Prokopenko, 128/Julia Sudnitskaya, 131/Nataliya Arzamasova, 132/MShev, 134/Tom Nance, 137/SARYMSAKOV ANDREY, 138/Sergiy Zavgorodny, 152/Nataliia K, 164/Nik Merkulov, 172/T. Dallas, 176/Filip Warulik, 180/Cipariss, 185/Kittibowornphatnon, 186/Geo-grafika, 193/anakondasp, 215 (above)/ Evgeny Kabardin, 215 (below)/ Olga Popova, 216 (above)/Binh Thanh Bui, 224 (above)/JIANG HONGYAN, 236 (below)/Serhii Tsyhanok, 239 (left)/jocic, 239 (right)/Galyasa,

Disclaimer: The author and publisher have endeavoured to contact all copyright holders. If any images used in this book have been reproduced without permission, we would like to rectify this in future editions and encourage owners of copyright not acknowledged to contact us at info@hbgi.ie.